CONTENTS

INTRODUCTION

The Ninja Foodi Digital Air Fryer Oven is more than just an electric oven; it's a multi-purpose device that offers 8 different programmable cooking functions.

You can now say goodbye to your toaster, oven, fryer, because with this high technology device you won't need them anymore.

Are you still wondering if buy this fantastic product or not? I will help you by giving you 5 reasons why you want Ninja Foodi Digital Air Fryer Oven in your kitchen:

1.   Healthier meals.

With this incredible cooking appliance you won't need to use much (or any) oil to get your food crispy and browned. This device is ideal for making fresh and frozen fries, onion rings, mozzarella sticks, chicken wings etc... You will finally enjoy your favourite food without getting concerned about your health.

2.   Cook fast and efficiently.

It will take just 60 second to preheat and most of the heat stays inside. Food cooks faster than in the oven or the stove, because the heat is not lost in the surrounding air. Ninja Foodi Digital Air Fryer Oven won't heat up your house in the summer like all the traditional ovens, and the cost of the electricity used is just pennies.

3.   Versatility.

As previously mentioned with this fantastic digital air fryer oven you can cook many different things in various ways. It really is more than just an oven!

4.   Space – Saving.

When the oven is not in use, you can simply flip it up and away to store. You can get your counter space freed with just a flip.

5.   Easy to use.

With Ninja Foodi Digital Air Fryer Oven, the only thing that you'll need to do is to put your food in the oven, set cooking function, the time and the temperature and then you will be free to walk away. It is so easy to use that you could teach your kids to use it for making after school snacks or quick lunches!

Ninja Foodi Digital Air Fryer Oven will revolutionize your way of cooking by saving time, money and space in your kitchen. Moreover, you will be always able to eat testy and healthy food anytime, anywhere.

The Ninja® Foodì Digital Air Fry Oven

The Ninja Foodi Digital Air Fryer Oven is a smart cooking device that has revolutionized the way of cooking. This cooking appliance is a first of its kind type of Air Fry Oven from Ninja, which has features not found in other Air Fryer Ovens, together with its unique design.

When you will unbox the Ninja Foodi Digital Air Fryer Oven, you will find a rectangular unit with 19.7" width x 7.5" height x 15.1" depth. It contains a flip lid and control panel on the front. The Air Fryer basket, sheet pan, and crumb tray are removable, and they all are dishwasher safe.

The crumb tray is placed inside and at the bottom of the oven to prevent the food drippings from falling on the oven base. The sheet pan is used for baking, broiling, or toasting. Whereas the Air fryer basket is used to evenly air fry the food. The wire rack can also be used for roasting purposes.

The control panel has an LED screen on its top, and it shows the timer in hours and minutes; and temperature in Fahrenheit. This screen also lit "PRE" in red colour to show if the device is preheating and "HOT" to show if the appliance should be left for cooling. Once it cools down, the LED shows the "FLIP" sign to indicate that it is ready to be flipped in its vertical storage position.

The modes and functions of the oven are listed below the Led screen. By rotating the dial, the user can switch from one mode to another, and a blue light will appear on one side of the selected mode. The power key is used to switch on and off the device, whereas Temp and Time buttons are used to adjust the temperature and time as well to select the number of slices and darkness of the toasts while toasting.

There is a light bulb fixed inside the oven, which can be switch ON/OFF using the light button on the control panel. It will enable the users to check the doneness of the food while it is cooked inside.

This product is a revolutionary kitchen appliance, because it can be used in 8 different ways:
- Air fry
- Air roast
- Air broil
- Bake
- Dehydrate
- Keep warm
- Toast
- Bagel

One small device that contains all these functions will save you time, money and space in your kitchen. When you are done using it, you can easily store it away by just flipping it up against your backsplash, which it can be done very easily. With this multi-functional device you can get extra-large capacity without sacrificing counter space with its unique and modern design.

The Ninja Foodi Digital Air Fryer Oven it has become very popular thanks to its diverse benefits, which you will find listed below:
- **Multi – purpose device** - as I previously mentioned, this unique and small device can be used for air roasting, air frying, baking, toasting bread and bagel, broil food and dehydrate. You will able to do all this, just by pushing one button that will also give you the possibility to switch the cooking mode while using it.
- **Flip up to store** - unlike the others electric ovens, The Ninja Foodi Digital Air Fryer Oven can help you to spare some space in your kitchen when not in use. How? Just by simply flipping the oven up and away to store. By putting it vertically, you will get more space on your kitchen shelf. In fact it takes up 50% less space when you flip it up and away to store against your backsplash.

- **Toaster function** - yes, it an oven that works as a toaster as well. On the control panel you will find 2 options for toasting (bread and bagel): you will select "bagel" if you want to toast some bagels or simply "toast" if you want to toast some bread slices. You will be able to fit and toast up to 9 slices of bread at a time, in this way, no one will be waiting for their toasts to be done. Press the "time/slice" button and then turn the dial to choose the number of slices that you would like to toast. Press "temp/darkness" button and choose the level of darkness/lightness for your bread slices. You can get crispy dark brown, golden brown or even soft light brown toasts as you desire.

- **Cook fast and evenly** – its unique design promotes speed and even cooking results. One of the most interesting features is that it can preheat in 60 seconds and it cooks up to 60% faster than a traditional oven with Air Roast. Moreover, you will be able to cook family – sized meals in as little as 20 minutes. It does up to 40% more even baking compared to similar products. Capacity wise, The Ninja Foodi Digital Air Fryer Oven, has a 45% larger pan cooking area, compared to appliances with flat surface. You will be able to fit a 13-inch pizza, 9 slices of toasts and 6 chicken breasts (6-8 oz. each).

- **Healthier food** – whit the Air Frying function, you will get your food with 75% less fat compared to the traditional frying methods. This has been tested either for hand-cut and deep-fried French fries.

- **Clean easily and efficiently** – the cleaning and maintenance of this fantastic smart kitchen device is effortless. A removable back panel allows you to easily access the interior for deep cleaning. It won't be necessary to spend extra money in cleaning chemicals, but will be enough a cloth and a mild soapy water. In case you want to put the removable parts in the dishwasher, you can, because they are dishwasher safe.

- **User-friendly** – all the features, including the control panel, are very easy to understand and to use. All buttons are cleared marked for each and single function. The main dial will allows you to switch from one mode to another and to decrease or increase the temperature and the cooking time. You can press these same dial for pausing or starting a function. Moreover, in the display, will also appear when the device has completing the cooling down procedure and the oven is ready to be flipped up.

- **High technology device** – due to its Digital Crisp Control Technology, this smart appliance include a precision-controlled temperature, heat source and air flow for ultimate versatility and optimum cooking performance.

The Ninja Foodi Air Fry oven is easily on its online stores, and this countertop convection oven comes with following features and accessories:

- **Ninja Air Fry Oven 1750-watt unit**
- **Wire rack (chrome plated)**
- **Sheet pan, 13x 13 inches, dishwasher safe**
- **Crumb tray (removable)**
- **Air fry basket, 13x 13 inches, dishwasher safe**

BREAKFAST AND BRUNCH RECIPES

Spinach & Tomato Frittata

Servings: 6
Cooking Time: 30 Minutes

Ingredients:

- 10 large eggs
- Salt and freshly ground black pepper, to taste
- 1 (5-ounce) bag baby spinach
- 2 cups grape tomatoes, halved
- 4 scallions, sliced thinly
- 8 ounces feta cheese, crumbled
- 3 tablespoons hot olive oil

Directions:

1. In a bowl, place the eggs, salt and black pepper and beat well.
2. Add the spinach, tomatoes, scallions and feta cheese and gently stir to combine.
3. Spread the oil in a baking pan and top with the spinach mixture.
4. Press "Power Button" of Ninja Foodi Digital Air Fry Oven and turn the dial to select "Air Bake" mode.
5. Press "Time Button" and again turn the dial to set the cooking time to 30 minutes.
6. Now push "Temp Button" and rotate the dial to set the temperature at 350 degrees F.
7. Press "Start/Pause" button to start.
8. When the unit beeps to show that it is preheated, open the lid.
9. Arrange pan over the wire rack and insert in the oven.
10. When cooking time is complete, open the lid and place the pan aside for about 5 minutes.
11. Cut into equal-sized wedges and serve hot.
12. Serving Suggestions: Enjoy your frittata with garlicky potatoes.
13. Variation Tip: Pick the right cheese for frittata.

Nutrition Info: Calories: 298 Fat: 23.6g Sat Fat: 9.3g Carbohydrates: 6.1g Fiber: 1.5g Sugar: 4.1g Protein: 17.2g

Potato Rosti

Servings: 2
Cooking Time: 15 Minutes

Ingredients:

- ½ pound potatoes, peeled, grated and squeezed
- ½ tablespoon fresh rosemary, chopped finely
- ½ tablespoon fresh thyme, chopped finely
- 1/8 teaspoon red pepper flakes, crushed
- Salt and ground black pepper, as required
- 2 tablespoons butter, softened

Directions:

1. In a bowl, mix together the potato, herbs, red pepper flakes, salt and black pepper.
2. Press "Power Button" of Ninja Foodi Digital Air Fry Oven and turn the dial to select the "Air Fry" mode.
3. Press the Time button and again turn the dial to set the cooking time to 15 minutes.
4. Now push the Temp button and rotate the dial to set the temperature at 355 degrees F.
5. Press "Start/Pause" button to start.
6. When the unit beeps to show that it is preheated, open the lid and lightly, grease the sheet pan.
7. Arrange the potato mixture into the "Sheet Pan" and shape it into an even circle.
8. Insert the "Sheet Pan" in the oven.
9. Cut the potato rosti into wedges.
10. Top with the butter and serve immediately.

Nutrition Info: Calories 185 Total Fat 11.8 g Saturated Fat 7.4 g Cholesterol 31 mg Sodium 167 mg Total Carbs 18.9 g Fiber 3.4 g Sugar 1.3 g Protein 2.1 g

Eggs In Avocado Cups

Servings: 2

Cooking Time: 10 Minutes

Ingredients:

- 1 avocado, halved and pitted
- 2 large eggs
- Salt and freshly ground black pepper, to taste
- 2 cooked bacon slices, crumbled

Directions:

1. Carefully scoop out about 2 teaspoons of flesh from each avocado half.
2. Crack 1 egg in each avocado half and sprinkle with salt and black pepper lightly.
3. Arrange avocado halves onto the greased piece of foil-lined sheet pan.
4. Press "Power Button" of Ninja Foodi Digital Air Fry Oven and turn the dial to select "Air Roast" mode.
5. Press "Time Button" and again turn the dial to set the cooking time to 10 minutes.
6. Now push "Temp Button" and rotate the dial to set the temperature at 375 degrees F.
7. Press "Start/Pause" button to start.
8. When the unit beeps to show that it is preheated, open the lid and insert the sheet pan in the oven.
9. When cooking time is complete, open the lid and transfer the avocado halves onto serving plates.
10. Top each avocado half with bacon pieces and serve.
11. Serving Suggestions: Serve these avocado halves with cherry tomatoes and fresh spinach.
12. Variation Tip: Smoked salmon can be replaced with bacon too.

Nutrition Info: Calories: 300 Fat: 26.6g Sat Fat: 6.4g Carbohydrates: 9g Fiber: 6.7g Sugar: 0.9g Protein: 9.7g

Sweet Potato Tots

Servings: 4

Cooking Time: 1 Hour

Ingredients:

- 1 tablespoon of potato starch
- 2 small sweet potatoes, peeled
- 1-1/4 teaspoons kosher salt
- 1/8 teaspoon of garlic powder
- ¾ cup ketchup

Directions:

1. Boil water in a medium-sized pot over high heat.
2. Add the potatoes. Cook till it becomes tender. Transfer them to a plate for cooling. Grate them in a mid-sized bowl.
3. Toss gently with garlic powder, 1 teaspoon of salt, and potato starch.
4. Shape the mix into tot-shaped cylinders.
5. Apply cooking spray on the air fryer basket.
6. Place half of the tots in a later in your basket. Apply some cooking spray.
7. Cook till it becomes light brown at 400°F.
8. Take out from the frying basket. Sprinkle some salt.
9. Serve with ketchup immediately.

Nutrition Info: Calories 80, Carbohydrates 19g, Total Fat 0g, Protein 1g, Fiber 2g, Sodium 335mg, Sugars 8g

Breakfast Frittata

Servings: 2

Cooking Time: 20 Minutes

Ingredients:

- 4 eggs, beaten lightly
- 4 oz. sausages, cooked and crumbled
- 1 onion, chopped
- 2 tablespoons of red bell pepper, diced
- ½ cup shredded Cheddar cheese

Directions:

1. Bring together the cheese, eggs, sausage, onion, and bell pepper in a bowl.
2. Mix well.
3. Preheat your air fryer to 180 degrees C or 360 degrees F.
4. Apply cooking spray lightly.
5. Keep your egg mix in a prepared cake pan.
6. Now cook in your air fryer till the frittata has become set.

Nutrition Info: Calories 487, Carbohydrates 3g, Cholesterol 443mg, Total Fat 39g, Protein 31g, Fiber 0.4g, Sodium 694mg, Sugars 1g

Tex-mex Hash Browns

Servings: 4

Cooking Time: 30 Minutes

Ingredients:

- 1-1/2 24 oz. potatoes, cut and peeled
- 1 onion, cut into small pieces
- 1 tablespoon of olive oil
- 1 jalapeno, seeded and cut
- 1 red bell pepper, seeded and cut

Directions:

1. Soak the potatoes in water.
2. Preheat your air fryer to 160 degrees C or 320 degrees F.
3. Drain and dry the potatoes using a clean towel.
4. Keep in a bowl.
5. Drizzle some olive oil over the potatoes, coat well.
6. Transfer to the air frying basket.
7. Add the onion, jalapeno, and bell pepper in the bowl.
8. Sprinkle half teaspoon olive oil, pepper, and salt. Coat well by tossing.
9. Now transfer your potatoes to the bowl with the veg mix from your fryer.
10. Place the empty basket into the air fryer. Raise the temperature to 180 degrees C or 356 degrees F.
11. Toss the contents of your bowl for mixing the potatoes with the vegetables evenly.
12. Transfer mix into the basket.
13. Cook until the potatoes have become crispy and brown.

Nutrition Info: Calories 197, Carbohydrates 34g, Cholesterol 0mg, Total Fat 5g, Protein 4g, Fiber 5g, Sodium 79mg, Sugars 3g

Cinnamon And Sugar Doughnuts

Servings: 9

Cooking Time: 16 Minutes

Ingredients:

- 1 teaspoon cinnamon
- 1/3 cup of white sugar
- 2 large egg yolks
- 2-1/2 tablespoons of butter, room temperature
- 1-1/2 teaspoons baking powder
- 2-1/4 cups of all-purpose flour

Directions:

1. Take a bowl and press your butter and white sugar together in it.
2. Add the egg yolks. Stir till it combines well.
3. Now sift the baking powder, flour, and salt in another bowl.
4. Keep one-third of the flour mix and half of the sour cream into your egg-sugar mixture. Stir till it combines well.
5. Now mix the remaining sour cream and flour. Refrigerate till you can use it.
6. Bring together the cinnamon and one-third sugar in your bowl.
7. Roll half-inch-thick dough.
8. Cut large slices (9) in this dough. Create a small circle in the center. This will make doughnut shapes.
9. Preheat your fryer to 175 degrees C or 350 degrees F.
10. Brush melted butter on both sides of your doughnut.
11. Keep half of the doughnuts in the air fryer's basket.
12. Apply the remaining butter on the cooked doughnuts.
13. Dip into the sugar-cinnamon mix immediately.

Nutrition Info: Calories 336, Carbohydrates 44g, Cholesterol 66mg, Total Fat 16g, Protein 4g, Fiber 1g, Sodium 390mg, Sugars 19g

Egg & Spinach Tart

Servings: 4

Cooking Time: 25 Minutes

Ingredients:

- 1 puff pastry sheet, trimmed into a 9x13-inch rectangle
- 4 eggs
- ½ cup cheddar cheese, grated
- 7 cooked thick-cut bacon strips
- ½ cup cooked spinach
- 1 egg, lightly beaten

Directions:

1. Arrange the pastry in a lightly greased "Sheet Pan".
2. With a small knife gently, cut a 1-inch border around the edges of the puff pastry without cutting all the way through.
3. With a fork, pierce the center of pastry a few times.
4. Press "Power Button" of Ninja Foodi Digital Air Fry Oven and turn the dial to select the "Air Bake" mode.
5. Press the Time button and again turn the dial to set the cooking time to 10 minutes.
6. Now push the Temp button and rotate the dial to set the temperature at 400 degrees F.
7. Press "Start/Pause" button to start.
8. When the unit beeps to show that it is preheated, open the lid.
9. Insert the "Sheet Pan" in the oven.
10. Remove the "Sheet Pan" from oven and sprinkle the cheese over the center.
11. Place the spinach and bacon in an even layer across the tart.
12. Now, crack the eggs, leaving space between each one.
13. Press "Power Button" of Ninja Foodi Digital Air Fry Oven and turn the dial to select the "Air Bake" mode.
14. Press the Time button and again turn the dial to set the cooking time to 15 minutes.
15. Now push the Temp button and rotate the dial to set the temperature at 400 degrees F.
16. Press "Start/Pause" button to start.
17. When the unit beeps to show that it is preheated, open the lid.
18. Insert the "Sheet Pan" in the oven.
19. Remove the "Sheet Pan" from oven and set aside to cool for 2-3 minutes before cutting.
20. With a pizza cutter, cut into4 portions and serve.

Nutrition Info: Calories 231 Total Fat 17.4 g Saturated Fat 8.2 g Cholesterol 236 mg Sodium 403 mg Total Carbs 5.7 g Fiber 0.3 g Sugar 0.8 g Protein 13.8 g

Roasted Cauliflower

Servings: 2

Cooking Time: 15 Minutes

Ingredients:

- 4 cups of cauliflower florets
- 1 tablespoon peanut oil
- 3 cloves garlic
- ½ teaspoon smoked paprika
- ½ teaspoon of salt

Directions:

1. Preheat your air fryer to 200 degrees C or 400 degrees F.
2. Now cut the garlic into half. Use a knife to smash it.
3. Keep in a bowl with salt, paprika, and oil.
4. Add the cauliflower. Coat well.
5. Transfer the coated cauliflower to your air fryer.
6. Cook for 10 minutes. Shake after 5 minutes.

Nutrition Info: Calories 136, Carbohydrates 12g, Cholesterol 0mg, Total Fat 8g, Protein 4g, Fiber 5.3g, Sodium 642mg, Sugars 5g

Eggs With Chicken

Servings: 3
Cooking Time: 12 Minutes

Ingredients:

- 4 large eggs, divided
- 2 tablespoons heavy cream
- Salt and ground black pepper, as required
- 2 teaspoons unsalted butter, softened
- 2 ounces cooked chicken, chopped
- 3 tablespoons Parmesan cheese, grated finely
- 2 teaspoons fresh parsley, minced

Directions:

1. In a bowl, add 1 egg, cream, salt and black pepper and beat until smooth.
2. In the bottom of a pie pan, place the butter and spread evenly.
3. In the bottom of pie pan, place chicken over butter and top with the egg mixture evenly.
4. Carefully, crack the remaining eggs on top.
5. Sprinkle with salt and black pepper and top with cheese and parsley evenly.
6. Press "Power Button" of Ninja Foodi Digital Air Fry Oven and turn the dial to select the "Air Fry" mode.
7. Press the Time button and again turn the dial to set the cooking time to 12 minutes.
8. Now push the Temp button and rotate the dial to set the temperature at 320 degrees F.
9. Press "Start/Pause" button to start.
10. When the unit beeps to show that it is preheated, open the lid.
11. Arrange pan over the "Wire Rack" and insert in the oven.
12. Cut into equal-sized wedges and serve hot.
13. Serve hot.

Nutrition Info: Calories 199 Total Fat 14.7 g Saturated Fat 6.7 g Cholesterol 287 mg Sodium 221 mg Total Carbs 0.8 g Fiber 0 g Sugar 0.5 g Protein 16.1 g

Eggs In Bread Cups

Servings: 4

Cooking Time: 23 Minutes

Ingredients:

- 4 bacon slices
- 2 bread slices, crust removed
- 4 eggs
- Salt and freshly ground black pepper, to taste

Directions:

1. Grease 4 cups of a muffin tin and set aside.
2. Heat a small frying pan over medium-high heat and cook the bacon slices for about 2-3 minutes.
3. With a slotted spoon, transfer the bacon slice onto a paper towel-lined plate to cool.
4. Break each bread slice in half.
5. Arrange 1 bread slices half in each of the prepared muffin cup and press slightly.
6. Now, arrange 1 bacon slice over each bread slice in a circular shape.
7. Crack 1 egg into each muffin cup and sprinkle with salt and black pepper.
8. Press "Power Button" of Ninja Foodi Digital Air Fry Oven and turn the dial to select "Air Bake" mode.
9. Press "Time Button" and again turn the dial to set the cooking time to 20 minutes.
10. Now push "Temp Button" and rotate the dial to set the temperature at 350 degrees F.
11. Press "Start/Pause" button to start.
12. When the unit beeps to show that it is preheated, open the lid.
13. Arrange the muffin tin over the wire rack and insert in the oven.
14. When cooking time is complete, open the lid and place the muffin tin onto a wire rack for about 10 minutes.
15. Serve warm.
16. Serving Suggestions: Feel free to top the bread cups with fresh herbs of your choice before serving.
17. Variation Tip: Pancetta can be used instead of bacon.

Nutrition Info: Calories: 98 Fat: 6.6g Sat Fat: 2.1g Carbohydrates: 2.6g Fiber: 0.1g Sugar: 0.5g Protein: 7.3g

Loaded Potatoes

Servings: 2

Cooking Time: 15 Minutes

Ingredients:

- 11 oz. baby potatoes
- 2 cut bacon slices
- 1-1/2 oz. low-fat cheddar cheese, shredded
- 1 teaspoon of olive oil
- 2 tablespoons low-fat sour cream

Directions:

1. Toss the potatoes with oil.
2. Place them in your air fryer basket. Cook till they get tender at 350°F. stir occasionally.
3. Cook the bacon meanwhile in a skillet till it gets crispy.
4. Take out the bacon from your pan. Crumble.
5. Keep the potatoes on a serving plate. Crush them lightly to split.
6. Top with cheese, chives, salt, crumbled bacon, and sour cream.

Nutrition Info: Calories 240, Carbohydrates 26g, Total Fat 12g, Protein 7g, Fiber 4g, Sodium 287mg, Sugars 3g

Baked Eggs

Servings: 4

Cooking Time: 12 Minutes

Ingredients:

- 1 cup marinara sauce, divided
- 1 tablespoon capers, drained and divided
- 8 eggs
- ¼ cup whipping cream, divided
- ¼ cup Parmesan cheese, shredded and divided
- Salt and ground black pepper, as required

Directions:

1. Grease 4 ramekins. Set aside.
2. Divide the marinara sauce in the bottom of each prepared ramekin evenly and top with capers.
3. Carefully, crack 2 eggs over marinara sauce into each ramekin and top with cream, followed by the Parmesan cheese.
4. Sprinkle each ramekin with salt and black pepper.
5. Press "Power Button" of Ninja Foodi Digital Air Fry Oven and turn the dial to select the "Air Bake" mode.
6. Press the Time button and again turn the dial to set the cooking time to 12 minutes.
7. Now push the Temp button and rotate the dial to set the temperature at 400 degrees F.
8. Press "Start/Pause" button to start.
9. When the unit beeps to show that it is preheated, open the lid.
10. Arrange the ramekins over the "Wire Rack" and insert in the oven.
11. Serve warm.

Nutrition Info: Calories 223 Total Fat 14.1 g Saturated Fat 5.5 g Cholesterol 341 mg Sodium 569 mg Total Carbs 9.8 g Fiber 1.7 g Sugar 6.2 g Protein 14.3 g

Sausage Patties

Servings: 4

Cooking Time: 10 Minutes

Ingredients:

- 1 pack sausage patties
- 1 serving cooking spray

Directions:

1. Preheat your air fryer to 200 degrees C or 400 degrees F.
2. Keep the sausage patties in a basket. Work in batches if needed.
3. Cook for 3 minutes.
4. Turn the sausage over and cook for another 2 minutes.

Nutrition Info: Calories 168, Carbohydrates 1g, Cholesterol 46mg, Total Fat 12g, Protein 14g, Fiber 0g, Sodium 393mg, Sugars 1g

FISH & SEAFOOD RECIPES

Fish Sticks

Servings: 4
Cooking Time: 10 Minutes

Ingredients:
- 16 oz. fillets of tilapia or cod
- 1 egg
- ¼ cup all-purpose flour
- ¼ cup Parmesan cheese, grated
- 1 teaspoon of paprika
- ½ cup bread crumbs

Directions:
1. Preheat your air fryer to 200 degrees C or 400 degrees F.
2. Use paper towels to pat dry your fish.
3. Cut into 1 x 3-inch sticks.
4. Keep flour in a dish. Beat the egg in another dish.
5. Bring together the paprika, cheese, bread crumbs and some pepper in another shallow dish.
6. Coat the sticks of fish in flour.
7. Now dip them in the egg and coat the bread crumbs mix.
8. Apply cooking spray on the air fryer basket.
9. Keep the sticks in your basket. They shouldn't touch.
10. Apply cooking spray on each fish stick.
11. Cook in the air fryer for 3 minutes. Flip over and cook for another 2 minutes.

Nutrition Info: Calories 217, Carbohydrates 17g, Cholesterol 92mg, Total Fat 5g, Protein 26g, Fiber 0.7g, Sugar 0g, Sodium 245mg

Green Beans With Southern Catfish

Servings: 2

Cooking Time: 10 Minutes

Ingredients:

- 2 catfish fillets
- ¾ oz. green beans, trimmed
- 1 large egg, beaten lightly
- 2 tablespoons of mayonnaise
- 1 teaspoon light brown sugar
- 1/3 cup breadcrumbs
- ½ teaspoon of apple cider vinegar

Directions:

1. Keep the green beans in a bowl. Apply cooking spray liberally.
2. Sprinkle some brown sugar, a pint of salt, and crushed red pepper (optional).
3. Keep in your air fryer basket. Cook at 400 degrees F until it becomes tender and brown.
4. Transfer to your bowl. Use aluminum foil to cover.
5. Toss the catfish in flour. Shake off the excesses.
6. Dip the pieces into the egg. Coat all sides evenly. Sprinkle breadcrumbs.
7. Keep fish in the fryer basket. Apply cooking spray.
8. Now cook at 400 degrees F until it is cooked thoroughly and brown.
9. Sprinkle pepper and ¼ teaspoon of salt.
10. Whisk together the vinegar, sugar, and mayonnaise in a bowl.
11. Serve the fish with tartar sauce and green beans.

Nutrition Info: Calories 562, Carbohydrates 31g, Total Fat 34g, Protein 33g, Fiber 7g, Sugar 16g, Sodium 677mg

Halibut & Shrimp With Pasta

Servings: 4
Cooking Time: 10 Minutes

Ingredients:

- 14 ounces pasta
- 4 tablespoons pesto, divided
- 4 (4-ounce) halibut steaks
- 2 tablespoons olive oil
- ½ pound tomatoes, chopped
- 8 large shrimp, peeled and deveined
- 2 tablespoons fresh lime juice
- 2 tablespoons fresh dill, chopped

Directions:

1. In the bottom of a baking pan, spread 1 tablespoon of pesto.
2. Place halibut steaks and tomatoes over pesto in a single layer and drizzle with the oil.
3. Now, place the shrimp on top in a single layer.
4. Drizzle with lime juice and sprinkle with dill.
5. Press "Power Button" of Ninja Foodi Digital Air Fry Oven and turn the dial to select "Air Fry" mode.
6. Press "Time Button" and again turn the dial to set the cooking time to 8 minutes.
7. Now push "Temp Button" and rotate the dial to set the temperature at 390 degrees F.
8. Press "Start/Pause" button to start.
9. When the unit beeps to show that it is preheated, open the lid.
10. Place the pan over the wire rack and insert in the oven.
11. Meanwhile, in a large pan of salted boiling water, add the pasta and cook for about 8-10 minutes or until desired doneness.
12. Drain the pasta and transfer into a large bowl.
13. Add the remaining pesto and toss to coat well.
14. When cooking time is complete, open the lid and divide the pasta onto serving plates.
15. Top with the fish mixture and serve immediately.
16. Serving Suggestions: Serve with the topping of freshly grated Parmesan.
17. Variation Tip: Linguine pasta will be the best choice for this recipe.

Nutrition Info: Calories: 606 Fat: 19.4g Sat Fat: 3.2g Carbohydrates: 59.1g Fiber: 1.1g Sugar: 2.5g Protein: 47.4g

Buttered Salmon

Servings: 2

Cooking Time: 10 Minutes

Ingredients:

- 2 (6-ounce) salmon fillets
- Salt and freshly ground black pepper, to taste
- 1 tablespoon butter, melted

Directions:

1. Season each salmon fillet with salt and black pepper and then, coat with the butter.
2. Press "Power Button" of Ninja Foodi Digital Air Fry Oven and turn the dial to select "Air Fry" mode.
3. Press "Time Button" and again turn the dial to set the cooking time to 10 minutes.
4. Now push "Temp Button" and rotate the dial to set the temperature at 360 degrees F.
5. Press "Start/Pause" button to start.
6. When the unit beeps to show that it is preheated, open the lid and grease the air fry basket.
7. Arrange the salmon fillets into the prepared air fry basket and insert in the oven.
8. When cooking time is complete, open the lid and transfer the salmon fillets onto serving plates.
9. Serve hot.
10. Serving Suggestions: Enjoy with roasted parsnip puree.
11. Variation Tip: Salmon should look bright and shiny.

Nutrition Info: Calories: 276 Fat: 16.3g Sat Fat: 5.2g Carbohydrates: 0g Fiber: 0g Sugar: 0g Protein: 33.1g

Grilled Fish Fillet In Pesto Sauce

Servings: 2

Cooking Time: 8 Minutes

Ingredients:

- 2 fish fillets, white fish
- 1 tablespoon of olive oil
- 2 cloves of garlic
- 1 bunch basil
- 1 tablespoon Parmesan cheese, grated

Directions:

1. Heat your air fryer to 180 degrees C.
2. Brush oil on your fish fillets. Season with salt and pepper.
3. Keep in your basket and into the fryer.
4. Cook for 6 minutes.
5. Keep the basil leaves with the cheese, olive oil, and garlic in your food processor.
6. Pulse until it becomes a sauce. Include salt to taste.
7. Keep fillets on your serving plate. Serve with pesto sauce.

Nutrition Info: Calories 1453, Carbohydrates 3g, Cholesterol 58mg, Total Fat 141g, Protein 43g, Fiber 1g, Sugar 0g, Sodium 1773mg

Spiced Tilapia

Servings: 2
Cooking Time: 12 Minutes

Ingredients:

- ¼ teaspoon garlic powder
- ¼ teaspoon onion powder
- ¼ teaspoon ground cumin
- Salt and ground black pepper, as required
- 2 (6-ounce) tilapia fillets
- 1 tablespoon butter, melted

Directions:

1. In a small bowl, mix together the spices, salt and black pepper.
2. Coat the tilapia fillets with oil and then rub with spice mixture.
3. Press "Power Button" of Ninja Foodi Digital Air Fry Oven and turn the dial to select the "Air Fry" mode.
4. Press the Time button and again turn the dial to set the cooking time to 12 minutes.
5. Now push the Temp button and rotate the dial to set the temperature at 360 degrees F.
6. Press "Start/Pause" button to start.
7. When the unit beeps to show that it is preheated, open the lid.
8. Arrange the tilapia fillets over the greased "Wire Rack" and insert in the oven.
9. Flip the tilapia fillets once halfway through.
10. Serve hot.

Nutrition Info: Calories 194 Total Fat 7.4 g Saturated Fat 4.3 g Cholesterol 98 mg Sodium 179 mg Total Carbs 0.6 g Fiber 0.1 g Sugar 0.2 g Protein 31.8 g

Blackened Fish Tacos

Servings: 4

Cooking Time: 15 Minutes

Ingredients:

- 1 oz. fillets of tilapia
- 1 can black beans, rinsed and drained
- 1 tablespoon olive oil
- 2 corn ears, cut the kernels
- 4 corn tortillas
- ¼ cup blackened seasoning

Directions:

1. Preheat your oven to 200 degrees C or 400 degrees F.
2. Bring together the corn, black beans, olive oil and salt in your bowl.
3. Stir gently until the corn and beans are coated evenly. Set aside.
4. Keep the fillets of fish on a work surface. Use paper towels to pat dry.
5. Apply cooking spray on each fillet lightly.
6. Sprinkle half of the blackened seasoning on the top.
7. Now flip over the fillets. Apply the cooking spray. Sprinkle the seasoning.
8. Keep the fish in your air fryer basket, in one single layer.
9. Cook for 2-3 minutes. Flip over and cook for another 2 minutes.
10. Take out and place on a plate.
11. Keep the corn and bean mix in the air fryer basket.
12. Cook for 8 minutes. Stir after 4 minutes.
13. Keep your fish in the corn tortillas. Apply the corn and bean mix on top.

Nutrition Info: Calories 376, Carbohydrates 43g, Cholesterol 42mg, Total Fat 8g, Protein 33g, Sugar 2g, Fiber 11g, Sodium 2210mg

Herbed Scallops

Servings: 2

Cooking Time: 14 Minutes

Ingredients:
- ¾ pound sea scallops, cleaned and pat dry
- 1 tablespoon butter, melted
- ¼ tablespoon fresh thyme, minced
- ¼ tablespoon fresh rosemary, minced
- Salt and freshly ground black pepper, to taste

Directions:
1. In a large bowl, place the scallops, butter, herbs, salt, and black pepper and toss to coat well.
2. Press "Power Button" of Ninja Foodi Digital Air Fry Oven and turn the dial to select "Air Fry" mode.
3. Press "Time Button" and again turn the dial to set the cooking time to 4 minutes.
4. Now push "Temp Button" and rotate the dial to set the temperature at 390 degrees F.
5. Press "Start/Pause" button to start.
6. When the unit beeps to show that it is preheated, open the lid and grease the air fry basket.
7. Arrange the scallops into the air fry basket and insert in the oven.
8. When cooking time is complete, open the lid and transfer the scallops onto serving plates.
9. Serve hot.
10. Serving Suggestions: Potato fries will be great with these scallops.
11. Variation Tip: Remove the side muscles from the scallops.

Nutrition Info: Calories: 203 Fat: 7.1g Sat Fat: 3.8g Carbohydrates: 4.5g Fiber: 0.3g Sugar: 0g Protein: 28.7g

Crusted Salmon

Servings: 2
Cooking Time: 15 Minutes

Ingredients:

- 2 (6-ounce) skinless salmon fillets
- Salt and ground black pepper, as required
- 3 tablespoons walnuts, chopped finely
- 3 tablespoons quick-cooking oats, crushed
- 2 tablespoons olive oil

Directions:

1. Rub the salmon fillets with salt and black pepper evenly.
2. In a bowl, mix together the walnuts, oats and oil.
3. Arrange the salmon fillets onto the greased "Sheet Pan" in a single layer.
4. Place the oat mixture over salmon fillets and gently, press down.
5. Press "Power Button" of Ninja Foodi Digital Air Fry Oven and turn the dial to select the "Air Bake" mode.
6. Press the Time button and again turn the dial to set the cooking time to 15 minutes.
7. Now push the Temp button and rotate the dial to set the temperature at 400 degrees F.
8. Press "Start/Pause" button to start.
9. When the unit beeps to show that it is preheated, open the lid.
10. Insert the "Sheet Pan" in oven.
11. Serve hot.

Nutrition Info: Calories 446 Total Fat 31.9 g Saturated Fat 4 g Cholesterol 75 mg Sodium 153 mg Total Carbs 6.4 g Fiber 1.6 g Sugar 0.2 g Protein 36.8 g

Crusted Sole

Servings: 2
Cooking Time: 15 Minutes

Ingredients:

- 2 teaspoons mayonnaise
- 1 teaspoon fresh chives, minced
- 3 tablespoons Parmesan cheese, shredded
- 2 tablespoons panko breadcrumbs
- Salt and freshly ground black pepper, to taste
- 2 (4-ounce) sole fillets

Directions:

1. In a shallow dish, mix together the mayonnaise and chives.
2. In another shallow dish, mix together the cheese, breadcrumbs, salt and black pepper.
3. Coat the fish fillets with mayonnaise mixture and then roll in cheese mixture.
4. Arrange the sole fillets onto the greased sheet pan in a single layer.
5. Press "Power Button" of Ninja Foodi Digital Air Fry Oven and turn the dial to select "Air Bake" mode.
6. Press "Time Button" and again turn the dial to set the cooking time to 15 minutes.
7. Now push "Temp Button" and rotate the dial to set the temperature at 450 degrees F.
8. Press "Start/Pause" button to start.
9. When the unit beeps to show that it is preheated, open the lid and insert the sheet pan in the oven.
10. When cooking time is complete, open the lid and transfer the fish fillets onto serving plates.
11. Serve hot.
12. Serving Suggestions: Roasted potatoes make a great side for fish.
13. Variation Tip: If you want a gluten-free option then use pork rinds instead of breadcrumbs.

Nutrition Info: Calories: 584 Fat: 14.6g Sat Fat: 5.2g Carbohydrates: 16.7g Fiber: 0.4g Sugar: 0.2g Protein: 33.2g

Lobster Tails With Garlic Butter-lemon

Servings: 2

Cooking Time: 10 Minutes

Ingredients:

- 2 lobster tails
- 1 teaspoon lemon zest
- 4 tablespoons of butter
- 1 garlic clove, grated
- 2 wedges of lemon

Directions:

1. Butterfly the lobster tails. Use kitchen shears to cut by length through the top shell's center and the meat.
2. Cut to the bottom portion of the shells.
3. Now spread halves of the tail apart.
4. Keep these tails in the basket of your air fry. The lobster meat should face up.
5. Melt the butter in your saucepan.
6. Add the garlic and lemon zest. Heat for 30 seconds.
7. Transfer two tablespoons of this mix to a bowl.
8. Brush on your lobster tails. Remove the remaining brushed butter.
9. Season with pepper and salt.
10. Cook in your air fryer at 195 degrees C or 380 degrees F. The lobster meat should turn opaque in about 5 or 7 minutes.
11. Apply the reserved butter over the lobster meat.
12. You can serve with lemon wedges.

Nutrition Info: Calories 462, Carbohydrates 3g, Cholesterol 129mg, Total Fat 42g, Protein 18g, Sugar 0g, Fiber 1g, Sodium 590mg

Buttered Trout

Servings: 2

Cooking Time: 10 Minutes

Ingredients:
- 2 (6-ounces) trout fillets
- Salt and ground black pepper, as required
- 1 tablespoon butter, melted

Directions:
1. Season each trout fillet with salt and black pepper and then, coat with the butter.
2. Arrange the trout fillets onto the greased "Sheet Pan" in a single layer.
3. Press "Power Button" of Ninja Foodi Digital Air Fry Oven and turn the dial to select the "Air Fry" mode.
4. Press the Time button and again turn the dial to set the cooking time to 10 minutes.
5. Now push the Temp button and rotate the dial to set the temperature at 360 degrees F.
6. Press "Start/Pause" button to start.
7. When the unit beeps to show that it is preheated, open the lid.
8. Insert the "Sheet Pan" in oven.
9. Flip the fillets once halfway through.
10. Serve hot.

Nutrition Info: Calories 374 Total Fat 20.2 g Saturated Fat 6.2 g Cholesterol 141 mg Sodium 232 mg Total Carbs 0 g Fiber 0 g Sugar 0 g Protein 45.4 g

Seasoned Catfish

Servings: 4

Cooking Time: 23 Minutes

Ingredients:

- 4 (4-ounce) catfish fillets
- 2 tablespoons Italian seasoning
- Salt and freshly ground black pepper, to taste
- 1 tablespoon olive oil
- 1 tablespoon fresh parsley, chopped

Directions:

1. Rub the fish fillets with seasoning, salt and black pepper generously and then coat with oil.
2. Press "Power Button" of Ninja Foodi Digital Air Fry Oven and turn the dial to select "Air Fry" mode.
3. Press "Time Button" and again turn the dial to set the cooking time to 20 minutes.
4. Now push "Temp Button" and rotate the dial to set the temperature at 400 degrees F.
5. Press "Start/Pause" button to start.
6. When the unit beeps to show that it is preheated, open the lid and grease the air fry basket.
7. Arrange the fish fillets into the prepared air fry basket and insert in the oven.
8. Flip the fish fillets once halfway through.
9. When cooking time is complete, open the lid and transfer the fillets onto serving plates.
10. Serve hot with the garnishing of parsley.
11. Serving Suggestions: Quinoa salad will be a great choice for serving.
12. Variation Tip: Season the fish according to your choice.

Nutrition Info: Calories: 205 Fat: 14.2g Sat Fat: 2.4g Carbohydrates: 0.8g Fiber: 0g Sugar: 0.6g Protein: 17.7g

Ranch Tilapia

Servings: 4

Cooking Time: 13 Minutes

Ingredients:

- ¾ cup cornflakes, crushed
- 1 (1-ounce) packet dry ranch-style dressing mix
- 2½ tablespoons vegetable oil
- 2 eggs
- 4 (6-ounce) tilapia fillets

Directions:

1. In a shallow bowl, crack the eggs and beat slightly.
2. In another bowl, add the cornflakes, ranch dressing, and oil and mix until a crumbly mixture forms.
3. Dip the fish fillets into egg and then, coat with the breadcrumbs mixture.
4. Press "Power Button" of Ninja Foodi Digital Air Fry Oven and turn the dial to select "Air Fry" mode.
5. Press "Time Button" and again turn the dial to set the cooking time to 13 minutes.
6. Now push "Temp Button" and rotate the dial to set the temperature at 356 degrees F.
7. Press "Start/Pause" button to start.
8. When the unit beeps to show that it is preheated, open the lid and grease the air fry basket.
9. Arrange the tilapia fillets into the prepared air fry basket and insert in the oven. When cooking time is complete, open the lid and transfer the fillets onto serving plates.
10. Serve hot.
11. Serving Suggestions: Serve tilapia with lemon butter.
12. Variation Tip: The skin should be removed, either before cooking or before serving.

Nutrition Info: Calories: 267 Fat: 12.2g Sat Fat: 3g Carbohydrates: 5.1g Fiber: 0.2g Sugar: 0.9g Protein: 34.9g

POULTRY RECIPES

Popcorn Chicken

Servings: 4
Cooking Time: 10 Minutes
Ingredients:
- 1 oz. chicken breast halves, boneless and skinless
- ½ teaspoon paprika
- ¼ teaspoon mustard, ground
- ¼ teaspoon of garlic powder
- 3 tablespoons of cornstarch

Directions:
1. Cut the chicken into small pieces and keep in a bowl.
2. Combine the paprika, garlic powder, mustard, salt, and pepper in another bowl.
3. Reserve a teaspoon of your seasoning mixture. Sprinkle the other portion on the chicken. Coat evenly by tossing.
4. Combine the reserved seasoning and cornstarch in a plastic bag.
5. Combine well by shaking.
6. Keep your chicken pieces in the bag. Seal it and shake for coating evenly.
7. Now transfer the chicken to a mesh strainer. Shake the excess cornstarch.
8. Keep aside for 5-10 minutes. The cornstarch should start to get absorbed into your chicken.
9. Preheat your air fryer to 200 degrees C or 390 degrees F.
10. Apply some oil on the air fryer basket.
11. Keep the chicken pieces inside. They should not overlap.
12. Apply cooking spray.
13. Cook until the chicken isn't pink anymore.

Nutrition Info: Calories 156, Carbohydrates 6g, Cholesterol 65mg, Total Fat 4g, Protein 24g, Sugar 0g, Fiber 0.3g, Sodium 493mg

Marinated Chicken Thighs

Servings: 4
Cooking Time: 30 Minutes
Ingredients:
- 4 (6-ounce) bone-in, skin-on chicken thighs
- Salt and freshly ground black pepper, to taste
- ½ cup Italian salad dressing
- 1 teaspoon onion powder
- 1 teaspoon garlic powder

Directions:
1. Season the chicken thighs with salt and black pepper evenly.
2. In a large bowl, add the chicken thighs and dressing and mix well.
3. Cover the bowl and refrigerate to marinate overnight.
4. Remove the chicken breast from the bowl and place onto a plate.
5. Sprinkle the chicken thighs with onion powder and garlic powder.
6. Press "Power Button" of Ninja Foodi Digital Air Fry Oven and turn the dial to select "Air Fry" mode.
7. Press "Time Button" and again turn the dial to set the cooking time to 30 minutes.
8. Now push "Temp Button" and rotate the dial to set the temperature at 360 degrees F.
9. Press "Start/Pause" button to start.
10. When the unit beeps to show that it is preheated, open the lid and grease the air fry basket.
11. Arrange the chicken thighs into the prepared basket and insert in the oven.
12. After 15 minutes of cooking, flip the chicken thighs once.
13. When cooking time is complete, open the lid and transfer the chicken thighs onto serving plates.
14. Serve hot.
15. Serving Suggestions: Enjoy with honey glazed baby carrots.
16. Variation Tip: Select the chicken thighs with a pinkish hue.

Nutrition Info: Calories: 413 Fat: 21g Sat Fat: 4.8g Carbohydrates: 4.1g Fiber: 0.1g Sugar: 2.8g Protein: 49.5g

Herbed Turkey Breast

Servings: 6
Cooking Time: 40 Minutes

Ingredients:

- ¼ cup unsalted butter, softened
- 2 tablespoons fresh rosemary, chopped
- 2 tablespoon fresh thyme, chopped
- 2 tablespoons fresh sage, chopped
- 2 tablespoons fresh parsley, chopped
- Salt and freshly ground black pepper, to taste
- 1 (4-pound) bone-in, skin-on turkey breast
- 2 tablespoons olive oil

Directions:

1. In a bowl, add the butter, herbs, salt and black pepper and mix well.
2. Rub the herb mixture under skin evenly.
3. Coat the outside of turkey breast with oil.
4. Place the turkey breast into the greased baking pan.
5. Press "Power Button" of Ninja Foodi Digital Air Fry Oven and turn the dial to select "Air Bake" mode.
6. Press "Time Button" and again turn the dial to set the cooking time to 40 minutes.
7. Now push "Temp Button" and rotate the dial to set the temperature at 350 degrees F.
8. Press "Start/Pause" button to start.
9. When the unit beeps to show that it is preheated, open the lid and insert baking pan in the oven.
10. When cooking time is complete, open the lid and place the turkey breast onto a platter for about 5-10 minutes before slicing.
11. With a sharp knife, cut the turkey breast into desired sized slices and serve.
12. Serving Suggestions: Roasted potatoes will accompany this turkey breast nicely.
13. Variation Tip: Use unsalted butter.

Nutrition Info: Calories: 333 Fat: 37g Sat Fat: 12.4g Carbohydrates: 1.8g Fiber: 1.1g Sugar: 0.1g Protein: 65.1g

Air Fryer Egg Rolls

Servings: 16

Cooking Time: 15 Minutes

Ingredients:

- 1 pack of egg roll wrappers
- 2 cups corn, thawed
- 1 can spinach, drained
- 1 can black beans, drained and rinsed
- 1 cup cheddar cheese, shredded

Directions:

1. Mix the corn, spinach, beans, Cheddar cheese, salt, and pepper in a bowl. This is for the filling.
2. Keep an egg roll wrapper.
3. Moisten lightly all the edges with your finger.
4. Keep a fourth of the filling at the wrapper's center.
5. Now fold a corner over the filling. Tuck the sides in to create a roll.
6. Repeat this process with the other wrappers.
7. Apply cooking spray on the egg rolls.
8. Preheat your air fryer at 199 degrees C or 390 degrees F.
9. Keep your egg rolls in its basket. They should not touch each other.
10. Fry for 7 minutes. Flip and cook for another 4 minutes.

Nutrition Info: Calories 260, Carbohydrates 27g, Cholesterol 25mg, Total Fat 12g, Protein 11g, Sugar 1g, Fiber 4g, Sodium 628mg

Thyme Duck Breast

Servings: 2
Cooking Time: 20 Minutes

Ingredients:

- 1 cup beer
- 1 tablespoon olive oil
- 1 teaspoon mustard
- 1 tablespoon fresh thyme, chopped
- Salt and freshly ground black pepper, to taste
- 1 (10½-ounce) duck breast

Directions:

1. In a bowl, add the beer, oil, mustard, thyme, salt, and black pepper and mix well
2. Add the duck breast and coat with marinade generously.
3. Cover and refrigerate for about 4 hours.
4. Arrange the duck breast onto the greased sheet pan.
5. Press "Power Button" of Ninja Foodi Digital Air Fry Oven and turn the dial to select "Air Fry" mode.
6. Press "Time Button" and again turn the dial to set the cooking time to 20 minutes.
7. Now push "Temp Button" and rotate the dial to set the temperature at 390 degrees F.
8. Press "Start/Pause" button to start.
9. When the unit beeps to show that it is preheated, open the lid and insert the sheet pan in the oven.
10. Flip the duck breast once halfway through.
11. When cooking time is complete, open the lid and place the duck breast onto a cutting board for about 5 minutes before slicing.
12. With a sharp knife, cut the duck breast into desired size slices and serve.
13. Serving Suggestions: Duck meat goes really well with caramelized onions or balsamic reduction.
14. Variation Tip: Look for a plump, firm breast for best flav

Nutrition Info: Calories: 315 Fat: 13.5g Sat Fat: 1.1g Carbohydrates: 5.7g Fiber: 0.7g Sugar: 0.1g Protein: 33.8g

Seasoned Chicken Tenders

Servings: 2

Cooking Time: 10 Minutes

Ingredients:

- 8 ounces chicken tenders
- 1 teaspoon BBQ seasoning
- Salt and ground black pepper, as required

Directions:

1. Line the "Sheet Pan" with a lightly, greased piece of foil.
2. Set aside.
3. Season the chicken tenders with BBQ seasoning, salt and black pepper.
4. Arrange the chicken tenders onto the prepared "Sheet Pan" in a single layer.
5. Press "Power Button" of Ninja Foodi Digital Air Fry Oven and turn the dial to select the "Air Bake" mode.
6. Press the Time button and again turn the dial to set the cooking time to 10 minutes.
7. Now push the Temp button and rotate the dial to set the temperature at 450 degrees F.
8. Press "Start/Pause" button to start.
9. When the unit beeps to show that it is preheated, open the lid and insert "Sheet Pan" in the oven.
10. Serve hot.

Nutrition Info: Calories 220 Total Fat 8.4 g Saturated Fat 2.3 g Cholesterol 101 mg Sodium 315 mg Total Carbs 0.5 g Fiber 0 g Sugar 0 g Protein 32.8 g

Peruvian Chicken Drumsticks & Green Crema

Servings: 6

Cooking Time: 15 Minutes

Ingredients:

- 6 chicken drumsticks
- 2 garlic cloves, grated
- 1 tablespoon of olive oil
- 1 tablespoon honey
- 1 cup of baby spinach leaves, with stems removed
- ¼ cup cilantro leaves
- ¾ cup of sour cream

Directions:

1. Bring together the honey, garlic, pepper, and salt in a bowl.
2. Add the drumsticks. Coat well by tossing.
3. Keep the drumsticks in a vertical position in the basket. Keep them leaning against the wall of the basket.
4. Cook in your air fryer at 200 degrees C or 400 degrees F for 15 minutes.
5. In the meantime, combine the sour cream, cilantro leaves, pepper and salt in a food processor bowl.
6. Process until the crema has become smooth.
7. Drizzle the crema sauce over your drumsticks.

Nutrition Info: Calories 337, Carbohydrates 6g, Cholesterol 82mg, Total Fat 25g, Protein 22g, Sugar 3g, Fiber 0.5g, Sodium 574mg

Spiced Chicken Thighs

Servings: 4
Cooking Time: 20 Minutes
Ingredients:
- 1 teaspoon ground cumin
- 1 teaspoon garlic powder
- ½ teaspoon smoked paprika
- ½ teaspoon ground coriander
- Salt and ground black pepper, as required
- 4 (5-ounce) chicken thighs

Directions:
1. In a large bowl, add the spices, salt and black pepper and mix well.
2. Coat the chicken thighs with oil and then rub with spice mixture.
3. Arrange the chicken thighs onto the sheet pan.
4. Press "Power Button" of Ninja Foodi Digital Air Fry Oven and turn the dial to select "Air Fry" mode.
5. Press "Time Button" and again turn the dial to set the cooking time to 20 minutes.
6. Now push "Temp Button" and rotate the dial to set the temperature at 400 degrees F.
7. Press "Start/Pause" button to start.
8. When the unit beeps to show that it is preheated, open the lid and insert the sheet pan in the oven.
9. Flip the chicken thighs once halfway through.
10. When cooking time is complete, open the lid and transfer the chicken thighs onto serving plates.
11. Serve hot.
12. Serving Suggestions: Serve with a fresh green salad.
13. Variation Tip: Adjust the ratio of spices according to your spice tolerance.
Nutrition Info: Calories: 334 Fat: 17.7g Sat Fat: 3.9g Carbohydrates: 0.9g Fiber: 0.2g Sugar: 0.2g Protein: 41.3g

Olive-brined Turkey Breast

Servings: 14

Cooking Time: 20 Minutes

Ingredients:

- 3-1/2 oz. turkey breasts, boneless and skinless
- ½ cup buttermilk
- ¾ cup olive brine
- 2 sprigs of thyme
- 1 rosemary sprig

Directions:

1. Bring together the buttermilk and olive brine.
2. Keep the turkey breast in a plastic bag. Pour the buttermilk-brine mix into this.
3. Add the thyme sprigs and rosemary.
4. Seal and bag. Keep it refrigerated.
5. Take it out after 8 hours. Set it aside and wait for it to reach room temperature.
6. Preheat your air fryer to 175 degrees C or 350 degrees F.
7. Cook the turkey breast for 12 minutes.
8. Flip over and cook for another 5 minutes. The turkey's center shouldn't be pink.

Nutrition Info: Calories 133, Carbohydrates 1g, Cholesterol 82mg, Total Fat 1g, Protein 30g, Sugar 0g, Fiber 0.6g, Sodium 62mg

Hard-boiled Eggs

Servings: 6

Cooking Time: 16 Minutes

Ingredients:

- 6 eggs, large

Directions:

1. Keep the eggs on your air fryer's wire rack.
2. Set the temperature to 250.
3. Take out the eggs once they are done.
4. Place them in a bowl with ice water.
5. Peel them off and serve.

Nutrition Info: Calories 91, Carbohydrates 1g, Total Fat 7g, Protein 6g, Sugar 0g, Fiber 0g, Sodium 62mg

Air Fryer Chicken Wings

Servings: 4

Cooking Time: 30 Minutes

Ingredients:

- 1-1/2 oz. chicken wings
- 1 teaspoon garlic powder
- 1 teaspoon kosher salt
- 1 tablespoon of butter, unsalted and melted
- ½ cup hot sauce

Directions:

1. Keep your chicken wings in 1 layer. Use paper towels to pat them dry.
2. Sprinkle garlic powder and salt evenly.
3. Now keep these wings in your air fryer at 380°F.
4. Cook for 20 minutes. Toss after every 5 minutes. The wings should be cooked through and tender.
5. Bring up the temperature to 400 degrees F.
6. Cook for 5-8 minutes until it has turned golden brown and crispy.
7. Toss your wings with melted butter (optional) before serving.

Nutrition Info: Calories 291, Carbohydrates 1g, Total Fat 23g, Protein 20g, Sugar 0.3g, Fiber 0g, Sodium 593mg

Nashville Chicken

Servings: 8

Cooking Time: 20 Minutes

Ingredients:

- 2 oz. chicken breast, boneless
- 2 tablespoons hot sauce
- ½ cup of olive oil
- 3 large eggs
- 3 cups all-purpose flour
- 1 teaspoon of chili powder
- 1-1/2 cups buttermilk

Directions:

1. Toss together the chicken, hot sauce, salt, and pepper in a bowl. Combine well.
2. Cover and refrigerate for three hours.
3. Pour flour into your bowl.
4. Now whisk the buttermilk and eggs together. Add 1 tablespoon of hot sauce.
5. For dredging your chicken, keep it in the flour first. Toss evenly for coating.
6. Keep it in your buttermilk mix. Then into the flour.
7. Keep them on your baking sheet.
8. Set the air fryer at 380 degrees. Place the tenders in your fryer.
9. Cook for 10 minutes.
10. For the sauce, whisk the spices and olive oil. Combine well.
11. Pour over the fried chicken immediately.

Nutrition Info: Calories 668, Carbohydrates 44g, Cholesterol 156mg, Total Fat 40g, Protein 33g, Sugar 5g, Fiber 2g, Sodium 847mg

Bacon-wrapped Chicken Breasts

Servings: 4

Cooking Time: 23 Minutes

Ingredients:

- 1 tablespoon palm sugar
- 6-7 Fresh basil leaves
- 2 tablespoons fish sauce
- 2 tablespoons water
- 2 (8-ounces) chicken breasts, cut each breast in half horizontally
- Salt and freshly ground black pepper, to taste
- 12 bacon strips
- 1½ teaspoon honey

Directions:

1. In a small heavy-bottomed pan, add palm sugar over medium-low heat and cook for about 2-3 minutes or until caramelized, stirring continuously.
2. Add the basil, fish sauce and water and stir to combine.
3. Remove from heat and transfer the sugar mixture into a large bowl.
4. Sprinkle each chicken breast with salt and black pepper.
5. Add the chicken pieces in the sugar mixture and coat generously.
6. Refrigerate to marinate for about 4-6 hours.
7. Wrap each chicken piece with 3 bacon strips.
8. Coat each piece with honey slightly.
9. Press "Power Button" of Ninja Foodi Digital Air Fry Oven and turn the dial to select "Air Fry" mode.
10. Press "Time Button" and again turn the dial to set the cooking time to 20 minutes.
11. Now push "Temp Button" and rotate the dial to set the temperature at 365 degrees F.
12. Press "Start/Pause" button to start.
13. When the unit beeps to show that it is preheated, open the lid and grease the air fry basket.
14. Arrange the chicken breasts into the prepared basket and insert in the oven.
15. Flip the chicken breasts once halfway through.
16. When cooking time is complete, open the lid and transfer the chicken breasts onto serving plates.
17. Serve hot.
18. Serving Suggestions: Serve with balsamic-glazed green beans.
19. Variation Tip: Use thick-cut bacon strips.

Nutrition Info: Calories: 709, Fat: 44.8g, Sat Fat: 14.3g, Carbohydrates: 6.8g, Fiber: 0g Sugar: 4.7g, Protein: 65.6g

Turkish Chicken Kebab

Servings: 4

Cooking Time: 15 Minutes

Ingredients:

- 1 oz. Chicken thighs, boneless and skinless
- ¼ cup Greek yogurt, plain
- 1 tablespoon tomato paste
- 1 tablespoon vegetable oil
- ½ teaspoon cinnamon, ground

Directions:

1. Stir together the tomato paste, Greek yogurt, oil, cinnamon, salt, and pepper in a bowl. The spices should blend well into the yogurt.
2. Cut the chicken into 4 pieces.
3. Now include your chicken pieces into the mixture. Make sure that the chicken is coated well with the mixture.
4. Refrigerate for 30 minutes' minimum.
5. Take out chicken from your marinade.
6. Keep in your air fryer basket in a single layer.
7. Set your fryer to 370 degrees F. Cook the chicken pieces for 8 minutes.
8. Flip over and cook for another 4 minutes.

Nutrition Info: Calories 375, Carbohydrates 4g, Cholesterol 112mg, Total Fat 31g, Protein 20g, Sugar 1g, Fiber 1g

MEAT RECIPES

Buttered Leg Of Lamb

Servings: 8

Cooking Time: 1¼ Hours

Ingredients:

- 1 (2¼-pound) boneless leg of lamb
- 3 tablespoons butter, melted
- Salt and freshly ground black pepper, to taste
- 4 fresh rosemary sprigs

Directions:

1. Rub the leg of lamb with butter and sprinkle with salt and black pepper.
2. Wrap the leg of lamb with rosemary sprigs.
3. Press "Power Button" of Ninja Foodi Digital Air Fry Oven and turn the dial to select "Air Fry" mode.
4. Press "Time Button" and again turn the dial to set the cooking time to 75 minutes.
5. Now push "Temp Button" and rotate the dial to set the temperature at 300 degrees F.
6. Press "Start/Pause" button to start.
7. When the unit beeps to show that it is preheated, open the lid and grease air fry basket.
8. Arrange the leg of lamb into the air fry basket and insert in the oven.
9. When cooking time is complete, open the lid and place the leg of lamb onto a cutting board for about 10 minutes before slicing.
10. Cut into desired sized pieces and serve.
11. Serving Suggestions: Dijon mustard glazed carrots will be great if served with le
12. Variation Tip: You can add spices of your choice for seasoning of the leg of lamb.

Nutrition Info: Calories: 278 Fat: 13.8g Sat Fat: 6.1g Carbohydrates: 0.5g Fiber: 0.4g Sugar: 0g Protein: 35.9g

Spiced Pork Shoulder

Servings: 6
Cooking Time: 55 Minutes
Ingredients:
- 1 teaspoon ground cumin
- 1 teaspoon cayenne pepper
- ½ teaspoon garlic powder
- ½ teaspoon onion powder
- Salt and ground black pepper, as required
- 2 pounds skin-on pork shoulder

Directions:
1. In a small bowl, place the spices, salt and black pepper and mix well.
2. Arrange the pork shoulder onto a cutting board, skin-side down.
3. Season the inner side of pork shoulder with salt and black pepper.
4. With kitchen twines, tie the pork shoulder into a long round cylinder shape.
5. Season the outer side of pork shoulder with spice mixture.
6. Press "Power Button" of Ninja Foodi Digital Air Fry Oven and turn the dial to select the "Air Roast" mode.
7. Press the Time button and again turn the dial to set the cooking time to 55 minutes.
8. Now push the Temp button and rotate the dial to set the temperature at 350 degrees F.
9. Press "Start/Pause" button to start.
10. When the unit beeps to show that it is preheated, open the lid and grease "Air Fry Basket".
11. Arrange the pork shoulder into "Air Fry Basket" and insert in the oven.
12. Remove from oven and place the pork shoulder onto a platter for about 10 minutes before slicing.
13. With a sharp knife, cut the pork shoulder into desired sized slices and serve.

Nutrition Info: Calories 445 Total Fat 32.5 g Saturated Fat 11.9 g Cholesterol 136 mg Sodium 131 mg Total Carbs 0.7 g Fiber 0.2 g Sugar 0.2 g Protein 35.4 g

Air-fried Meatloaf

Servings: 4
Cooking Time: 45 Minutes

Ingredients:

- 8 oz. pork, ground
- 8 oz. veal, ground
- 1 large egg
- ¼ cup bread crumbs
- 1.4 cup cilantro, chopped
- 1 teaspoon of olive oil
- 2 teaspoons chipotle chili sauce

Directions:

1. Preheat your air fryer to 200 degrees C or 400 degrees F.
2. Bring together the veal and pork in a baking dish. Make sure that it goes into your air fryer basket.
3. Create a well. Now add the cilantro, egg, bread crumbs, salt, and pepper.
4. Use your hands to mix well and create a loaf.
5. Combine the olive oil and chipotle chili sauce in a bowl. Whisk well.
6. Keep it aside.
7. Cook the meatloaf in your air fryer. Take it out and add the juicy mix.
8. Bring back the meatloaf to the fryer. Bake for 7 minutes.
9. Turn the fryer off. Allow the meatloaf to rest for 6 minutes inside.
10. Take it out and let it rest for 5 more minutes.
11. Slice before serving.

Nutrition Info: Calories 311, Carbohydrates 13g, Cholesterol 123mg, Total Fat 19g, Fiber 0.7g, Protein 22g, Sugar 8g, Sodium 536mg

Beef Kabobs

Servings: 4

Cooking Time: 10 Minutes

Ingredients:

- 1 oz. beef ribs, cut into small 1-inch pieces
- 2 tablespoons soy sauce
- 1/3 cup low-fat sour cream
- 1 bell pepper
- ½ onion

Directions:

1. Mix soy sauce and sour cream in a bowl.
2. Keep the chunks of beef in the bowl. Marinate for 30 minutes' minimum.
3. Now cut the onion and bell pepper into one-inch pieces.
4. Soak 8 skewers in water.
5. Thread the bell pepper, onions, and beef on the skewers. Add some pepper.
6. Cook for 10 minutes in your pre-heated air fryer. Turn after 5 minutes.

Nutrition Info: Calories 297, Carbohydrates 4g, Cholesterol 84mg, Total Fat 21g, Protein 23g, Sugar 2g, Sodium 609mg, Calcium 49mg

Pork Stuffed Bell Peppers

Servings: 4

Cooking Time: 1 Hour 10 Minutes

Ingredients:

- 4 medium green bell peppers
- 2/3-pound ground pork
- 2 cups cooked white rice
- 1½ cups marinara sauce, divided
- 1 teaspoon Worcestershire sauce
- 1 teaspoon Italian seasoning
- Salt and ground black pepper, as required
- ½ cup mozzarella cheese, shredded

Directions:

1. Cut the tops from bell peppers and then carefully remove the seeds.
2. Heat a large skillet over medium heat and cook the pork for bout 6-8 minutes, breaking into crumbles.
3. Add the rice, ¾ cup of marinara sauce, Worcestershire sauce, Italian seasoning, salt and black pepper and stir to combine.
4. Remove from the heat.
5. Arrange the bell peppers into the greased baking pan.
6. Carefully, stuff each bell pepper with the pork mixture and top each with the remaining sauce.
7. Press "Power Button" of Ninja Foodi Digital Air Fry Oven and turn the dial to select the "Air Bake" mode.
8. Press the Time button and again turn the dial to set the cooking time to 60 minutes.
9. Now push the Temp button and rotate the dial to set the temperature at 350 degrees F.
10. Press "Start/Pause" button to start.
11. When the unit beeps to show that it is preheated, open the lid.
12. Insert the baking pan in oven.
13. After 50 minutes of cooking, top each bell pepper with cheese.
14. Serve warm.

Nutrition Info: Calories 580 Total Fat 7.1 g Saturated Fat 2.2 g Cholesterol 60 mg Sodium 509 mg Total Carbs 96.4 g Fiber 5.2 g Sugar 14.8 g Protein 30.3 g

Glazed Pork Tenderloin

Servings: 3
Cooking Time: 20 Minutes
Ingredients:
- 2 tablespoons Sriracha
- 2 tablespoons maple syrup
- ¼ teaspoon red pepper flakes, crushed
- Salt, to taste
- 1 pound pork tenderloin

Directions:
1. In a small bowl, add the Sriracha, maple syrup, red pepper flakes and salt and mix well.
2. Brush the pork tenderloin with mixture evenly.
3. Press "Power Button" of Ninja Foodi Digital Air Fry Oven and turn the dial to select "Air Fry" mode.
4. Press "Time Button" and again turn the dial to set the cooking time to 20 minutes.
5. Now push "Temp Button" and rotate the dial to set the temperature at 350 degrees F.
6. Press "Start/Pause" button to start.
7. When the unit beeps to show that it is preheated, open the lid and grease air fry basket.
8. Arrange the pork tenderloin into the air fry basket and insert in the oven.
9. When cooking time is complete, open the lid and place the pork tenderloin onto a platter for about 10 minutes before slicing.
10. With a sharp knife, cut the roast into desired sized slices and serve.
11. Serving Suggestions: Fig and arugula salad will brighten the taste of tenderloin.
12. Variation Tip: The addition of dried herbs will add a delish touch in pork tenderloin.

Nutrition Info: Calories: 261 Fat: 5.4g Sat Fat: 1.8g Carbohydrates: 11g Fiber: 0g Sugar: 8g Protein: 39.6g

Lamb Sirloin Steak

Servings: 4
Cooking Time: 15 Minutes

Ingredients:

- 1 oz. lamb sirloin steaks, boneless
- 5 garlic cloves
- 1 teaspoon fennel, ground
- ½ onion
- 1 teaspoon cinnamon, ground

Directions:

1. Add all the ingredients in your blender bowl other than the lamb chops.
2. Pulse and blend until you see the onion minced fine. All the ingredients should be blended well.
3. Now keep your lamb chops in a big-sized bowl.
4. Slash the meat and fat with a knife.
5. The marinade should penetrate.
6. Include the spice paste. Mix well.
7. Refrigerate the mixture for half an hour.
8. Keep the steaks of lamb in your air fryer basket.
9. Cook, flipping once.

Nutrition Info: Calories 189, Carbohydrates 3g, Total Fat 9g, Protein 24g, Fiber 1g

Buttered Rib Eye Steak

Servings: 3
Cooking Time: 14 Minutes
Ingredients:
- 2 (8-ounce) rib eye steaks
- 2 tablespoons butter, melted
- Salt and ground black pepper, as required

Directions:
1. Coat the steak with butter and then, sprinkle with salt and black pepper evenly.
2. Press "Power Button" of Ninja Foodi Digital Air Fry Oven and turn the dial to select the "Air Roast" mode.
3. Press the Time button and again turn the dial to set the cooking time to 14 minutes.
4. Now push the Temp button and rotate the dial to set the temperature at 400 degrees F.
5. Press "Start/Pause" button to start.
6. When the unit beeps to show that it is preheated, open the lid and grease "Air Fry Basket".
7. Arrange the steaks into "Air Fry Basket" and insert in the oven.
8. Remove from the oven and place steaks onto a platter for about 5 minutes.
9. Cut each steak into desired size slices and serve.

Nutrition Info: Calories 388 Total Fat 23.7 g Saturated Fat 110.2 g Cholesterol 154 mg Sodium 278 mg Total Carbs 0 g Fiber 0 g Sugar 0 g Protein 41 g

Pork Skewers With Mango Salsa & Black Bean

Servings: 4

Cooking Time: 10 Minutes

Ingredients:

- 1 lb. pork tenderloin, cut into small cubes
- ½ can black beans, rinsed and drained
- 1 mango, peeled, seeded, and chopped
- 4-1/2 teaspoons of onion powder
- 4-1/2 teaspoons thyme, crushed
- 1 tablespoon vegetable oil
- ¼ teaspoon cloves, ground

Directions:

1. Stir in the thyme, onion powder, salt, and cloves in a bowl to create the seasoning mixture.
2. Keep a tablespoon of this for the pork. Transfer the remaining to an airtight container for later.
3. Preheat your air fryer to 175 degrees C or 350 degrees F.
4. Thread the chunks of pork into the skewers.
5. Brush oil on the pork. Sprinkle the seasoning mix on all sides.
6. Keep in your air fryer basket.
7. Cook for 5 minutes.
8. Mash one-third of the mango in your bowl in the meantime.
9. Stir the remaining mango in, and also salt, pepper, and black beans.
10. Serve the salsa with the pork skewers.

Nutrition Info: Calories 372, Carbohydrates 35g, Cholesterol 49mg, Total Fat 16g, Fiber 7g, Protein 22g, Sugar 18g, Sodium 1268mg

Almonds Crusted Rack Of Lamb

Servings: 5

Cooking Time: 35 Minutes

Ingredients:

- 1 tablespoon olive oil
- 1 garlic clove, minced
- Salt and freshly ground black pepper, to taste
- 1 (1¾-pound) rack of lamb
- 1 egg
- 1 tablespoon breadcrumbs
- 3 ounces almonds, finely chopped

Directions:

1. In a bowl, mix together the oil, garlic, salt, and black pepper.
2. Coat the rack of lamb evenly with oil mixture.
3. Crack the egg in a shallow bowl and beat well.
4. In another bowl, mix together the breadcrumbs and almonds.
5. Dip the rack of lamb in beaten egg and then, coat with almond mixture.
6. Press "Power Button" of Ninja Foodi Digital Air Fry Oven and turn the dial to select "Air Fry" mode.
7. Press "Time Button" and again turn the dial to set the cooking time to 30 minutes.
8. Now push "Temp Button" and rotate the dial to set the temperature at 220 degrees F.
9. Press "Start/Pause" button to start.
10. When the unit beeps to show that it is preheated, open the lid and grease air fry basket.
11. Place the rack of lamb into the prepared air fry basket and insert in the oven.
12. After 30 minutes, set the temperature of to 390 degrees F for 5 minutes.
13. When cooking time is complete, open the lid and place the rack of lamb onto a cutting board for about 5 minutes.
14. With a sharp knife, cut the rack of lamb into individual chops and serve.
15. Serving Suggestions: Serve with a fresh spinach salad.
16. Variation Tip: For best result, remove the silver skin from rack of lamb.

Nutrition Info: Calories: 408 Fat: 26.3g Sat Fat: 6.3g Carbohydrates: 4.9g Fiber: 2.2g Sugar: 0.9g Protein: 37.2g

Beef Sirloin Roast

Servings: 8
Cooking Time: 50 Minutes
Ingredients:
- 1 tablespoon smoked paprika
- 1 teaspoon ground cumin
- 1 teaspoon garlic powder
- Salt and freshly ground black pepper, to taste
- 2½ pounds sirloin roast

Directions:
1. In a bowl, mix together the spices, salt and black pepper.
2. Rub the roast with spice mixture generously.
3. Place the sirloin roast into the greased baking pan.
4. Press "Power Button" of Ninja Foodi Digital Air Fry Oven and turn the dial to select "Air Roast" mode.
5. Press "Time Button" and again turn the dial to set the cooking time to 50 minutes.
6. Now push "Temp Button" and rotate the dial to set the temperature at 350 degrees F.
7. Press "Start/Pause" button to start.
8. When the unit beeps to show that it is preheated, open the lid and insert baking pan in the oven.
9. When cooking time is complete, open the lid and place the roast onto a platter for about 10 minutes before slicing.
10. With a sharp knife, cut the beef roast into desired sized slices and serve.
11. Serving Suggestions: Serve this roast with a topping of herbed butter.
12. Variation Tip: Rub the seasoning over the roast with your fingers, covering the entire exterior with an even layer.

Nutrition Info: Calories: 260 Fat: 11.9g Sat Fat: 4.4g Carbohydrates: 0.4g Fiber: 0.1g Sugar: 0.1g Protein: 38g

Sweet Potato, Brown Rice, And Lamb

Servings: 2

Cooking Time: 10 Minutes

Ingredients:

- ¼ cup lamb, cooked and puréed
- ½ cup cooked brown rice
- ¼ cup of sweet potato purée

Directions:

1. Keep all the ingredients in your bowl.
2. Pulse until you achieve the desired consistency.
3. Process with milk to get a smoother consistency.
4. Store in an airtight container. Refrigerate.

Nutrition Info: Calories 37, Carbohydrates 5g, Cholesterol 7mg, Total Fat 1g, Protein 2g, Fiber 1g, Sodium 6mg

Simple Beef Tenderloin

Servings: 10

Cooking Time: 50 Minutes

Ingredients:

- 1 (3½-pound) beef tenderloin, trimmed
- 2 tablespoons olive oil
- Salt and ground black pepper, as required

Directions:

1. With kitchen twine, tie the tenderloin.
2. Rub the tenderloin with oil and season with salt and black pepper.
3. Place the tenderloin into the greased baking pan.
4. Press "Power Button" of Ninja Foodi Digital Air Fry Oven and turn the dial to select the "Air Roast" mode.
5. Press the Time button and again turn the dial to set the cooking time to 50 minutes.
6. Now push the Temp button and rotate the dial to set the temperature at 400 degrees F.
7. Press "Start/Pause" button to start.
8. When the unit beeps to show that it is preheated, open the lid and insert baking pan in the oven.
9. Remove from oven and place the tenderloin onto a platter for about 10 minutes before slicing.
10. With a sharp knife, cut the tenderloin into desired sized slices and serve.

Nutrition Info: Calories 351 Total Fat 17.3 g Saturated Fat 5.9 g Cholesterol 146 mg Sodium 109 mg Total Carbs 0 g Fiber 0 g Sugar 0 g Protein 46 g

Rosemary Garlic Lamb Chops

Servings: 2

Cooking Time: 12 Minutes

Ingredients:

- 4 chops of lamb
- 1 teaspoon olive oil
- 2 teaspoon garlic puree
- Fresh garlic
- Fresh rosemary

Directions:

1. Keep your lamb chops in the fryer grill pan.
2. Season the chops with pepper and salt. Brush some olive oil.
3. Add some garlic puree on each chop.
4. Cover the grill pan gaps with garlic cloves and rosemary sprigs.
5. Refrigerate the grill pan to marinate.
6. Take out after 1 hour. Keep in the fryer and cook for 5 minutes.
7. Use your spatula to turn the chops over.
8. Add some olive oil and cook for another 5 minutes.
9. Set aside for a minute.
10. Take out the rosemary and garlic before serving.

Nutrition Info: Calories 678, Carbohydrates 1g, Cholesterol 257mg, Total Fat 38g, Protein 83g, Sugar 0g, Sodium 200mg

VEGETARIAN AND VEGAN RECIPES

Spicy Green Beans

Servings: 4
Cooking Time: 25 Minutes

Ingredients:

- ¾ oz. green beans, trimmed
- 1 teaspoon of soy sauce
- 1 tablespoon sesame oil
- 1 garlic clove, minced
- 1 teaspoon of rice wine vinegar

Directions:

1. Preheat your air fryer to 200 degrees C or 400 degrees F.
2. Keep the green beans in a bowl.
3. Whisk together the soy sauce, sesame oil, garlic, and rice wine vinegar in another bowl.
4. Pour the green beans into it.
5. Coat well by tossing. Leave it for 5 minutes to marinate.
6. Transfer half of the beans to your air fryer basket.
7. Cook for 12 minutes. Shake the basket after 6 minutes.
8. Repeat with the other portion of green beans.

Nutrition Info: Calories 81, Carbohydrates 7g, Cholesterol 0mg, Total Fat 5g, Protein 2g, Sugar 1g, Fiber 3g, Sodium 80mg

Roasted Cauliflower And Broccoli

Servings: 6

Cooking Time: 15 Minutes

Ingredients:

- 3 cups cauliflower florets
- 3 cups of broccoli florets
- ¼ teaspoon of sea salt
- ½ teaspoon of garlic powder
- 2 tablespoons olive oil

Directions:

1. Preheat your air fryer to 200 degrees C or 400 degrees F.
2. Keep your florets of broccoli in a microwave-safe bowl.
3. Cook in your microwave for 3 minutes on high temperature. Drain off the accumulated liquid.
4. Now add the olive oil, cauliflower, sea salt, and garlic powder to the broccoli in the bowl.
5. Combine well by mixing.
6. Pour this mix now into your air fryer basket.
7. Cook for 10 minutes. Toss the vegetables after 5 minutes for even browning.

Nutrition Info: Calories 77, Carbohydrates 6g, Cholesterol 0mg, Total Fat 5g, Protein 2g, Sugar 2g, Fiber 3g, Sodium 103mg

Basil Tomatoes

Servings: 2

Cooking Time: 10 Minutes

Ingredients:

- 3 tomatoes, halved
- Olive oil cooking spray
- Salt and freshly ground black pepper, to taste
- 1 tablespoon fresh basil, chopped

Directions:

1. Drizzle the cut sides of the tomato halves with cooking spray evenly.
2. Then, sprinkle with salt, black pepper and basil.
3. Press "Power Button" of Ninja Foodi Digital Air Fry Oven and turn the dial to select "Air Fry" mode.
4. Press "Time Button" and again turn the dial to set the cooking time to 10 minutes.
5. Now push "Temp Button" and rotate the dial to set the temperature at 320 degrees F.
6. Press "Start/Pause" button to start.
7. When the unit beeps to show that it is preheated, open the lid.
8. Arrange the tomatoes into the air fry basket and insert in the oven.
9. When cooking time is complete, open the lid and transfer the tomatoes onto serving plates.
10. Serve warm.
11. Serving Suggestions: You can use these tomatoes in pasta and pasta salads with a drizzle of balsamic vinegar.
12. Variation Tip: Fresh thyme can also be used instead of basil.

Nutrition Info: Calories: 34 Fat: 0.4g Sat Fat: 0.1g Carbohydrates: 7.2g Fiber: 2.2g Sugar: 4.9g Protein: 1.7g

Tofu With Broccoli

Servings: 3
Cooking Time: 15 Minutes

Ingredients:

- 8 ounces firm tofu, drained, pressed and cubed
- 1 head broccoli, cut into florets
- 1 tablespoon butter, melted
- 1 teaspoon ground turmeric
- ¼ teaspoon paprika
- Salt and ground black pepper, as required

Directions:

1. In a bowl, mix together all ingredients.
2. Place the tofu mixture in the greased cooking pan.
3. Press "Power Button" of Ninja Foodi Digital Air Fry Oven and turn the dial to select the "Air Fry" mode.
4. Press the Time button and again turn the dial to set the cooking time to 15 minutes.
5. Now push the Temp button and rotate the dial to set the temperature at 390 degrees F.
6. Press "Start/Pause" button to start.
7. When the unit beeps to show that it is preheated, open the lid.
8. Insert the baking pan in oven.
9. Toss the tofu mixture once halfway through.
10. Serve hot.

Nutrition Info: Calories 119 Total Fat 7.4 g Saturated Fat 3.1 g Cholesterol 10 mg Sodium 115 mg Total Carbs 7.5 g Fiber 3.1 g Sugar 1.9 g Protein 8.7 g

Air Fryer Pumpkin Keto Pancakes

Servings: 2

Cooking Time: 5 Minutes

Ingredients:

- ½ cup pumpkin puree
- 1 teaspoon of vanilla extract
- 2 eggs
- ½ cup peanut butter
- ½ teaspoon baking soda

Directions:

1. Use parchment paper to line the basket of your air fryer.
2. Apply some cooking spray.
3. Bring together the eggs, peanut butter, pumpkin puree, baking soda, salt, and eggs in a bowl. Combine well by stirring.
4. Place 3 tablespoons of the batter in each pancake. There should be a half-inch space between them.
5. Keep the basket in your air fryer oven.
6. Cook for 4 minutes at 150 degrees C or 300 degrees F.

Nutrition Info: Calories 586, Carbohydrates 20g, Cholesterol 186mg, Total Fat 46g, Protein 23g, Sugar 9g, Fiber 6g, Sodium 906mg

Glazed Mushrooms

Servings: 4

Cooking Time: 15 Minutes

Ingredients:

- ¼ cup soy sauce
- ¼ cup honey
- ¼ cup balsamic vinegar
- 2 garlic cloves, chopped finely
- ½ teaspoon red pepper flakes, crushed
- 18 ounces fresh Cremini mushrooms, halved

Directions:

1. In a bowl, place the soy sauce, honey, vinegar, garlic and red pepper flakes and mix well. Set aside.
2. Place the mushroom into the greased baking pan in a single layer.
3. Press "Power Button" of Ninja Foodi Digital Air Fry Oven and turn the dial to select "Air Bake" mode.
4. Press "Time Button" and again turn the dial to set the cooking time to 15 minutes.
5. Now push "Temp Button" and rotate the dial to set the temperature at 350 degrees F.
6. Press "Start/Pause" button to start.
7. When the unit beeps to show that it is preheated, open the lid.
8. Insert the baking pan in oven.
9. After 8 minutes of cooking, place the honey mixture in baking pan and toss to coat well.
10. When cooking time is complete, open the lid and transfer the mushrooms onto serving plates.
11. Serve hot.
12. Serving Suggestions: Topping of fresh chives or marjoram gives a delish touch to mushrooms.
13. Variation Tip: Maple syrup will be an excellent substitute for honey.

Nutrition Info: Calories: 113 Fat: 0.2g Sat Fat: 0g Carbohydrates: 24.7g Fiber: 1g Sugar: 20g Protein: 4.4g

Garlicky Brussels Sprout

Servings: 4
Cooking Time: 15 Minutes

Ingredients:

- 1 pound Brussels sprouts, cut in half
- 2 tablespoons oil
- 2 garlic cloves, minced
- ¼ teaspoon red pepper flakes, crushed
- Salt and freshly ground black pepper, to taste

Directions:

1. In a bowl, add all the ingredients and toss to coat well.
2. Press "Power Button" of Ninja Foodi Digital Air Fry Oven and turn the dial to select "Air Fry" mode.
3. Press "Time Button" and again turn the dial to set the cooking time to 12 minutes.
4. Now push "Temp Button" and rotate the dial to set the temperature at 390 degrees F.
5. Press "Start/Pause" button to start.
6. When the unit beeps to show that it is preheated, open the lid.
7. Arrange the Brussels sprouts into the air fry basket and insert in the oven.
8. When cooking time is complete, open the lid and transfer the Brussels sprouts onto serving plates.
9. Serve hot.
10. Serving Suggestions: Sprinkle with flaky sea salt before serving.
11. Variation Tip: Look for small to medium sprouts for better taste.

Nutrition Info: Calories: 113 Fat: 9g Sat Fat: 1.3g Carbohydrates: 8.3g Fiber: 2.6g Sugar: 4.2g Protein: 2.8g

Fried Chickpeas

Servings: 4

Cooking Time: 20 Minutes

Ingredients:

- 1 can chickpeas, rinsed and drained
- 1 tablespoon olive oil
- 1 tablespoon of nutritional yeast
- 1 teaspoon garlic, granulated
- 1 teaspoon of smoked paprika

Directions:

1. Spread the chickpeas on paper towels. Cover using a second paper towel later.
2. Allow them to dry for half an hour.
3. Preheat your air fryer to 180 degrees C or 355 degrees F.
4. Bring together the nutritional yeast, chickpeas, smoked paprika, olive oil, salt, and garlic in a mid-sized bowl. Coat well by tossing.
5. Now add your chickpeas to the fryer.
6. Cook for 16 minutes until they turn crispy. Shake them in 4-minute intervals.

Nutrition Info: Calories 133, Carbohydrates 17g, Cholesterol 0mg, Total Fat 5g, Protein 5g, Sugar 0g, Fiber 4g, Sodium 501mg

Baked Potatoes

Servings: 2

Cooking Time: 1 Hour

Ingredients:

- 1 tablespoon peanut oil
- 2 large potatoes, scrubbed
- ½ teaspoon of coarse sea salt

Directions:

1. Preheat your air fryer to 200 degrees C or 400 degrees F.
2. Brush peanut oil on your potatoes.
3. Sprinkle some salt.
4. Keep them in the basket of your air fryer.
5. Cook the potatoes for an hour.

Nutrition Info: Calories 360, Carbohydrates 64g, Cholesterol 0mg, Total Fat 8g, Protein 8g, Sugar 3g, Fiber 8g, Sodium 462mg

Potato Gratin

Servings: 4

Cooking Time: 20 Minutes

Ingredients:

- 2 large potatoes, sliced thinly
- 5½ tablespoons cream
- 2 eggs
- 1 tablespoon plain flour
- ½ cup cheddar cheese, grated

Directions:

1. Press "Power Button" of Ninja Foodi Digital Air Fry Oven and turn the dial to select "Air Fry" mode.
2. Press "Time Button" and again turn the dial to set the cooking time to 10 minutes.
3. Now push "Temp Button" and rotate the dial to set the temperature at 355 degrees F.
4. Press "Start/Pause" button to start.
5. When the unit beeps to show that it is preheated, open the lid.
6. Arrange the potato slices in the air fry basket and insert in the oven.
7. Meanwhile, in a bowl, add cream, eggs and flour and mix until a thick sauce forms.
8. When cooking time is complete, open the lid and remove the potato slices from the basket.
9. Divide the potato slices in 4 ramekins evenly and top with the egg mixture evenly, followed by the cheese.
10. Press "Power Button" of Ninja Foodi Digital Air Fry Oven and turn the dial to select "Air Fry" mode.
11. Press "Time Button" and again turn the dial to set the cooking time to 10 minutes.
12. Now push "Temp Button" and rotate the dial to set the temperature at 390 degrees F.
13. Arrange the ramekins in the air fry basket and insert in the oven.
14. Press "Start/Pause" button to start.
15. When cooking time is complete, open the lid and remove the ramekins from the oven.
16. Serve warm.
17. Serving Suggestions: Serve this gratin with fresh lettuce.
18. Variation Tip: Make sure to cut the potato slices thinly.

Nutrition Info: Calories: 233 Fat: 8g Sat Fat: 4.3g Carbohydrates: 31.3g Fiber: 4.5g Sugar: 2.7g Protein: 9.7g

Potato-skin Wedges

Servings: 4
Cooking Time: 30 Minutes

Ingredients:

- 4 medium potatoes
- 3 tablespoons of canola oil
- 1 cup of water
- ¼ teaspoon black pepper, ground
- 1 teaspoon paprika

Directions:

1. Keep the potatoes in a big-sized pot. Add salted water and keep covered. Boil.
2. Bring down the heat to medium. Let it simmer. It should become tender.
3. Drain the water on.
4. Keep in a bowl and place in the refrigerator until it becomes cool.
5. Bring together the paprika, oil, salt, and black pepper in a bowl.
6. Now cut the potatoes into small quarters. Toss them into your mixture.
7. Preheat your air fryer to 200 degrees C or 400 degrees F.
8. Add half of the wedges of potato into the fryer basket. Keep them skin-down. Don't overcrowd.
9. Cook for 15 minutes. It should become golden brown.

Nutrition Info: Calories 276, Carbohydrates 38g, Cholesterol 0mg, Total Fat 12g, Protein 4g, Sugar 2g, Fiber 5g, Sodium 160mg

Roasted Okra

Servings: 1

Cooking Time: 15 Minutes

Ingredients:

- ½ oz. okra, trimmed ends and sliced pods
- ¼ teaspoon salt
- 1 teaspoon olive oil
- 1/8 teaspoon black pepper, ground

Directions:

1. Preheat your air fryer to 175 degrees C or 350 degrees F.
2. Bring together the olive oil, okra, pepper, and salt in a mid-sized bowl.
3. Stir gently.
4. Keep in your air fryer basket. It should be in one single layer.
5. Cook for 5 minutes in the fryer. Toss once and cook for another 5 minutes.
6. Toss once more. Cook again for 2 minutes.

Nutrition Info: Calories 138, Carbohydrates 16g, Cholesterol 0mg, Total Fat 6g, Protein 5g, Sugar 3g, Fiber 7g, Sodium 600mg

Spicy Butternut Squash

Servings: 4

Cooking Time: 20 Minutes

Ingredients:

- 1 medium butternut squash, peeled, seeded and cut into chunk
- 2 teaspoons cumin seeds
- 1/8 teaspoon garlic powder
- 1/8 teaspoon chili flakes, crushed
- Salt and freshly ground black pepper, to taste
- 1 tablespoon olive oil
- 2 tablespoons pine nuts
- 2 tablespoons fresh cilantro, chopped

Directions:

1. In a bowl, mix together the squash, spices, and oil.
2. Press "Power Button" of Ninja Foodi Digital Air Fry Oven and turn the dial to select "Air Fry" mode.
3. Press "Time Button" and again turn the dial to set the cooking time to 20 minutes.
4. Now push "Temp Button" and rotate the dial to set the temperature at 375 degrees F.
5. Press "Start/Pause" button to start.
6. When the unit beeps to show that it is preheated, open the lid and grease the air fry basket.
7. Arrange the squash chunks into the prepared air fry basket and insert in the oven.
8. When cooking time is complete, open the lid and transfer the squash chunks onto serving plates.
9. Serve hot with the garnishing of pine nuts and cilantro.
10. Serving Suggestions: Serve with a sprinkle of sweet dried cranberries.
11. Variation Tip: you can microwave the butternut squash for 2-3 mins to make it softer and easier to remove the skin.

Nutrition Info: Calories: 191 Fat: 7g Sat Fat: 0.8g Carbohydrates: 34.3g Fiber: 6g Sugar: 6.4g Protein: 3.7g

Veggie Kabobs

Servings: 6
Cooking Time: 10 Minutes
Ingredients:
- ¼ cup carrots, peeled and chopped
- ¼ cup French beans
- ½ cup green peas
- 1 teaspoon ginger
- 3 garlic cloves, peeled
- 3 green chilies
- ¼ cup fresh mint leaves
- ½ cup cottage cheese
- 2 medium boiled potatoes, mashed
- ½ teaspoon five-spice powder
- Salt, to taste
- 2 tablespoons corn flour
- Olive oil cooking spray

Directions:
1. In a food processor, add the carrot, beans, peas, ginger, garlic, mint, cheese and pulse until smooth.
2. Transfer the mixture into a bowl.
3. Add the mashed potatoes, five-spice powder, salt and corn flour and with your hands mix until well combined.
4. Shape the mixture into equal-sized small balls.
5. Press each ball around a skewer in a sausage shape.
6. Spray the skewers with cooking spray.
7. Press "Power Button" of Ninja Foodi Digital Air Fry Oven and turn the dial to select "Air Fry" mode.
8. Press "Time Button" and again turn the dial to set the cooking time to 10 minutes.
9. Now push "Temp Button" and rotate the dial to set the temperature at 390 degrees F.
10. Press "Start/Pause" button to start.
11. When the unit beeps to show that it is preheated, open the lid and grease the air fry basket.
12. Arrange the skewers into the prepared air fry basket and insert in the oven.
13. When cooking time is complete, open the lid and transfer the skewers onto a platter.
14. Serve warm.
15. Serving Suggestions: Enjoy these kabobs wt yogurt dip.
16. Variation Tip: You can add spices of your choice in these veggie kabobs

Nutrition Info: Calories: 120, Fat: 0.8g Sat Fat: 0.3g, Carbohydrates: 21.9g Fiber: 4.9g Sugar: 1.8g Protein: 6.3g

SNACK & DESSERT RECIPES

Spicy Chickpeas

Servings: 4
Cooking Time: 10 Minutes

Ingredients:

- 1 (15-ounce) can chickpeas, rinsed and drained
- 1 tablespoon olive oil
- ½ teaspoon cayenne pepper
- ½ teaspoon smoked paprika
- ½ teaspoon ground cumin
- 1/8 teaspoon ground cinnamon
- Salt, to taste

Directions:

1. In a bowl, add all the ingredients and toss to coat well.
2. Press "Power Button" of Ninja Foodi Digital Air Fry Oven and turn the dial to select "Air Fry" mode.
3. Press "Time Button" and again turn the dial to set the cooking time to 10 minutes.
4. Now push "Temp Button" and rotate the dial to set the temperature at 390 degrees F.
5. Press "Start/Pause" button to start.
6. When the unit beeps to show that it is preheated, open the lid.
7. Arrange the chickpeas into the air fry basket and insert in the oven.
8. When cooking time is complete, open the lid and transfer the chickpeas into a bowl.
9. Serve warm.
10. Serving Suggestions: These roasted chickpeas can also be used as a topping of potato soup.
11. Variation Tip: You can adjust the ratio of spices according to your taste.

Nutrition Info: Calories: 146 Fat: 4.5g Sat Fat: 0.5g Carbohydrates: 18.8g Fiber: 4.6g Sugar: 0.1g Protein: 6.3g

Jalapeño Poppers

Servings: 6
Cooking Time: 13 Minutes

Ingredients:

- 12 large jalapeño peppers
- 8 ounces cream cheese, softened
- ¼ cup scallion, chopped
- ¼ cup fresh cilantro, chopped
- ¼ teaspoon onion powder
- ¼ teaspoon garlic powder
- Salt, to taste
- 1/3 cup sharp cheddar cheese, grated

Directions:

1. Carefully cut off one-third of each pepper lengthwise and then scoop out the seeds and membranes.
2. In a bowl, mix together the cream cheese, scallion, cilantro, spices and salt.
3. Stuff each pepper with the cream cheese mixture and top with cheese.
4. Arrange the jalapeño peppers onto the greased sheet pan.
5. Press "Power Button" of Ninja Foodi Digital Air Fry Oven and turn the dial to select "Air Fry" mode.
6. Press "Time Button" and again turn the dial to set the cooking time to 13 minutes.
7. Now push "Temp Button" and rotate the dial to set the temperature at 400 degrees F.
8. Press "Start/Pause" button to start.
9. When the unit beeps to show that it is preheated, open the lid and insert the sheet pan in the oven.
10. When cooking time is complete, open the lid and transfer the jalapeño poppers onto a platter.
11. Serve immediately.
12. Serving Suggestions:
13. Variation Tip:

Nutrition Info: Calories: 171 Fat: 15.7g Sat Fat: 9.7g Carbohydrates: 3.7g Fiber: 1.3g Sugar: 1.2g Protein: 4.9g

Chicken Wings

Servings: 4
Cooking Time: 25 Minutes

Ingredients:

- 1½ pounds chicken wingettes and drumettes
- 1/3 cup tomato sauce
- 2 tablespoons balsamic vinegar
- 2 tablespoons maple syrup
- ½ teaspoon liquid smoke
- ¼ teaspoon red pepper flakes, crushed
- Salt, as required

Directions:

1. Arrange the wings onto the greased "Sheet Pan".
2. Place the tofu mixture in the greased "Sheet Pan".
3. Press "Power Button" of Ninja Foodi Digital Air Fry Oven and turn the dial to select the "Air Fry" mode.
4. Press the Time button and again turn the dial to set the cooking time to 25 minutes.
5. Now push the Temp button and rotate the dial to set the temperature at 380 degrees F.
6. Press "Start/Pause" button to start.
7. When the unit beeps to show that it is preheated, open the lid.
8. Insert the "Sheet Pan" in oven.
9. Meanwhile, in a small pan, add the remaining ingredients over medium heat and cook for about 10 minutes, stirring occasionally.
10. Remove from oven and place the chicken wings into a bowl.
11. Add the sauce and toss to coat well.
12. Serve immediately.

Nutrition Info: Calories 356 Total Fat 12.7 g Saturated Fat 3.5 g Cholesterol 151 mg Sodium 293 mg Total Carbs 7.9 g Fiber 0.3 g Sugar 6.9 g Protein 49.5 g

Buffalo Chicken Wings

Servings: 5

Cooking Time: 16 Minutes

Ingredients:

- 2 pounds frozen chicken wings, drums and flats separated
- 2 tablespoons olive oil
- 2-4 tablespoons Buffalo sauce
- ½ teaspoon red pepper flakes, crushed
- Salt, to taste

Directions:

1. Coat the chicken wings with oil evenly.
2. Press "Power Button" of Ninja Foodi Digital Air Fry Oven and turn the dial to select "Air Fry" mode.
3. Press "Time Button" and again turn the dial to set the cooking time to 16 minutes.
4. Now push "Temp Button" and rotate the dial to set the temperature at 390 degrees F.
5. Press "Start/Pause" button to start.
6. When the unit beeps to show that it is preheated, open the lid.
7. Arrange the chicken wings into the air fry basket and insert in the oven.
8. After 7 minutes, flip the wings.
9. Meanwhile, in a large bowl, add the Buffalo sauce, red pepper flakes and salt and mix well.
10. When cooking time is complete, open the lid.
11. Transfer the wings into the bowl of Buffalo sauce and toss to coat well.
12. Serve immediately.
13. Serving Suggestions: Serving with blue cheese dip enhances the taste of these wings.
14. Variation Tip: To avoid spiciness, add a little sweetener in the sauce mixture.

Nutrition Info: Calories: 394 Fat: 19.1g Sat Fat: 4.5g Carbohydrates: 0.2g Fiber: 0.1g Sugar: 0.1g Protein: 52.5g

Crispy Coconut Prawns

Servings: 4
Cooking Time: 12 Minutes

Ingredients:

- ½ cup flour
- ¼ teaspoon paprika
- Salt and freshly ground white pepper, to taste
- 2 egg whites
- ¾ cup panko breadcrumbs
- ½ cup unsweetened coconut, shredded
- 2 teaspoons lemon zest, grated finely
- 1 pound prawns, peeled and deveined

Directions:

1. In a shallow dish, place the flour, paprika, salt and white pepper and mix well.
2. In a second shallow dish, add the egg whites and beat lightly.
3. In a third shallow dish, place the breadcrumbs, coconut and lemon zest and mix well.
4. Coat the prawns with flour mixture, then dip into egg whites and finally coat with the coconut mixture.
5. Place the prawns in the greased sheet pan.
6. Press "Power Button" of Ninja Foodi Digital Air Fry Oven and turn the dial to select "Air Bake" mode.
7. Press "Time Button" and again turn the dial to set the cooking time to 12 minutes.
8. Now push "Temp Button" and rotate the dial to set the temperature at 400 degrees F.
9. Press "Start/Pause" button to start.
10. When the unit beeps to show that it is preheated, open the lid and insert the sheet pan in the oven.
11. Flip the prawns once halfway through.
12. When cooking time is complete, open the lid and transfer the prawns onto a platter.
13. Serve hot.
14. Serving Suggestions: Sweet chili sauce will accompany these prawns nicely.
15. Variation Tip: You may use regular breadcrumbs instead of panko.

Nutrition Info: Calories: 310 Fat: 6.9g Sat Fat: 4.1g Carbohydrates: 18.7g Fiber: 1.5g Sugar: 0.9g Protein: 3.2g

Chocolate Pudding

Servings: 4
Cooking Time: 12 Minutes
Ingredients:

- ½ cup butter
- 2/3 cup dark chocolate, chopped
- ¼ cup caster sugar
- 2 medium eggs
- 2 teaspoons fresh orange rind, finely grated
- ¼ cup fresh orange juice
- 2 tablespoons self-rising flour

Directions:

1. In a microwave-safe bowl, add the butter and chocolate and microwave on high heat for about 2 minutes or until melted completely, stirring after every 30 seconds.
2. Remove from the microwave and stir the mixture until smooth.
3. Add the sugar and eggs and whisk until frothy.
4. Add the orange rind and juice, followed by flour and mix until well combined.
5. Divide mixture into 4 greased ramekins about ¾ full.
6. Press "Power Button" of Ninja Foodi Digital Air Fry Oven and turn the dial to select "Air Fry" mode.
7. Press "Time Button" and again turn the dial to set the cooking time to 12 minutes.
8. Now push "Temp Button" and rotate the dial to set the temperature at 355 degrees F.
9. Press "Start/Pause" button to start.
10. When the unit beeps to show that it is preheated, open the lid.
11. Arrange the ramekins into the air fry basket and insert in the oven.
12. When cooking time is complete, open the lid and place the ramekins set aside to cool completely before serving.
13. Serving Suggestions: Serve with the garnishing of fresh strawberries and mint leaves.
14. Variation Tip: This pudding can be served chilled too.

Nutrition Info: Calories: 454 Fat: 33.6g Sat Fat: 21.1g Carbohydrates: 34.2g Fiber: 1.2g Sugar: 28.4g Protein: 5.7g

Gluten-free Cherry Crumble

Servings: 4

Cooking Time: 25 Minutes

Ingredients:

- 3 cups pitted cherries
- 2 teaspoons of lemon juice
- 1/3 cup butter
- 1 cup gluten-free all-purpose baking flour
- 1 teaspoon vanilla powder
- 10 tablespoons of white sugar

Directions:

1. Cube the butter and refrigerate for about 15 minutes. It should get firm.
2. Preheat your air fryer to 165 degrees C or 325 degrees F.
3. Bring together the pitted cherries, lemon juice, and 2 tablespoons of sugar in your bowl. Mix well.
4. Pour the cherry mix into a baking dish.
5. Now mix 6 tablespoons of sugar and flour in a bowl.
6. Use your fingers to cut in the butter. Particles should be pea-size.
7. Keep them over the cherries. Press down lightly.
8. Stir in the vanilla powder and 2 tablespoons of sugar in your bowl.
9. Dust the sugar topping over flour and cherries.
10. Transfer to your air fryer and bake.
11. Leave it inside for 10 minutes once the baking is done.
12. Set aside for 5 minutes to cool.

Nutrition Info: Calories 576, Carbohydrates 76g, Cholesterol 41mg, Total Fat 28g, Protein 5g, Sugar 49g, Fiber 6g, Sodium 109mg

Vanilla Cheesecake

Servings: 6

Cooking Time: 14 Minutes

Ingredients:

- 1 cup honey graham cracker crumbs
- 2 tablespoons unsalted butter, softened
- 1 pound cream cheese, softened
- ½ cup sugar
- 2 large eggs

Directions:

1. Line a round baking pan with parchment paper.
2. For crust: in a bowl, add the graham cracker crumbs and butter.
3. Place the crust into the baking dish and press to smooth.
4. Press "Power Button" of Ninja Foodi Air Fry Oven and turn the dial to select the "Air Fry" mode.
5. Press "Time Button" and again turn the dial to set the cooking time to 4 minutes.
6. Now push "Temp Button" and rotate the dial to set the temperature at 350 degrees F.
7. Press "Start/Pause" button to start.
8. When the unit beeps to show that it is preheated, open the lid.
9. Arrange the baking pan of crust into the air fry basket and insert in the oven.
10. When cooking time is complete, open the lid and place the crust aside to cool for about 10 minutes.
11. Meanwhile, in a bowl, add the cream cheese and sugar and whisk until smooth.
12. Now, place the eggs, one at a time and whisk until the mixture becomes creamy.
13. Add the vanilla extract and mix well.
14. Place the cream cheese mixture over the crust evenly.
15. Press "Power Button" of Ninja Foodi Air Fry Oven and turn the dial to select the "Air Fry" mode.
16. Press "Time Button" and again turn the dial to set the cooking time to 10 minutes.
17. Now push "Temp Button" and rotate the dial to set the temperature at 350 degrees F.
18. Press "Start/Pause" button to start.
19. When the unit beeps to show that it is preheated, open the lid.
20. Arrange the baking pan into the air fry basket and insert in the oven.
21. When cooking time is complete, open the lid and place the pan onto a wire rack to cool completely.
22. Refrigerate overnight before serving.
23. Serving Suggestions: Serve with the topping of fresh berries.
24. Variation Tip: Your cream cheese should always be at room temperature.

Nutrition Info: Calories: 470 Fat: 33.9g, Sat Fat: 20.6g Carbohydrates: 349g, Fiber: 0.5g Sugar: 22g Protein: 9.4g

Air Fryer Beignets

Servings: 7

Cooking Time: 15 Minutes

Ingredients:

- ½ cup all-purpose flour
- 1 egg, separated
- ½ teaspoon of baking powder
- 1-1/2 teaspoons melted butter
- ¼ cup white sugar
- ½ teaspoon of vanilla extract

Directions:

1. Preheat your air fryer to 185 degrees C or 370 degrees F.
2. Whisk together the sugar, flour, butter, egg yolk, vanilla extract, baking powder, salt, and water in a bowl. Combine well by stirring.
3. Use an electric hand mixer to beat the white portion of the egg in a bowl.
4. Fold this into the batter.
5. Now use a small ice cream scoop to add the mold.
6. Keep the mold into the air fryer basket.
7. Fry for 10 minutes in your air fryer.
8. Take out the mold and the pop beignets carefully.
9. Flip them over on a round of parchment paper.
10. Now transfer the parchment round with the beignets into the fryer basket.
11. Cook for 4 more minutes.

Nutrition Info: Calories 99, Carbohydrates 16g, Cholesterol 29mg, Total Fat 3g, Protein 2g, Sugar 9g, Fiber 0.2g, Sodium 74mg

Chocolate Mug Cake

Servings: 2

Cooking Time: 17 Minutes

Ingredients:

- ¼ cup flour
- 2 tablespoons sugar
- ¼ teaspoon baking powder
- 1/8 teaspoon baking soda
- 1/8 teaspoon salt
- 2 tablespoons milk
- 2 tablespoons applesauce
- ½ tablespoon vegetable oil
- ¼ teaspoon vanilla extract
- 2 tablespoons chocolate chips

Directions:

1. In a bowl, mix together the flour, sugar, baking powder, baking soda and salt.
2. Add the milk, applesauce, oil and vanilla extract and mix until well combined.
3. Gently, fold in the chocolate chips.
4. Place the mixture into an over proof mug.
5. Press "Power Button" of Ninja Foodi Digital Air Fry Oven and turn the dial to select "Air Bake" mode.
6. Press "Time Button" and again turn the dial to set the cooking time to 17 minutes.
7. Now push "Temp Button" and rotate the dial to set the temperature at 375 degrees F.
8. Press "Start/Pause" button to start.
9. When the unit beeps to show that it is preheated, open the lid.
10. Arrange the mug over the wire rack and insert in the oven.
11. When cooking time is complete, open the lid and place the mug onto a wire rack to cool for about 10 minutes.
12. Serve warm.
13. Serving Suggestions: Sprinkle the cake with powdered sugar before serving.
14. Variation Tip: Use the best quality chocolate chips for cake.

Nutrition Info: Calories: 204 Fat: 7g Sat Fat: 3.1g Carbohydrates: 33g Fiber: 1g Sugar: 19.8g Protein: 2.9g

CPSIA information can be obtained
at www.ICGtesting.com
Printed in the USA
LVHW020156050221
678443LV00009B/374

9 781922 547880